Handbook of HYDROTHERAPY

Basics of Hydrotherapy - A guide to BNYS students

DR. VRINDA BEDEKAR
BNYS, MS, MD

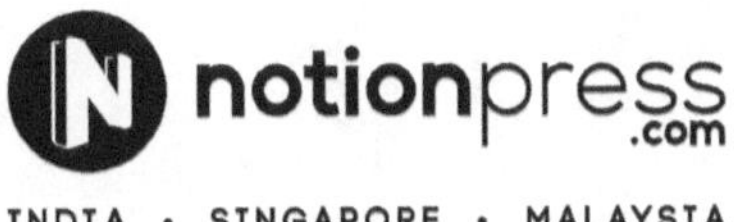

Copyright © Dr. Vrinda Bedekar 2024
All Rights Reserved.

ISBN 979-8-89632-405-8

This book has been published with all efforts taken to make the material error-free after the consent of the author. However, the author and the publisher do not assume and hereby disclaim any liability to any party for any loss, damage, or disruption caused by errors or omissions, whether such errors or omissions result from negligence, accident, or any other cause.

While every effort has been made to avoid any mistake or omission, this publication is being sold on the condition and understanding that neither the author nor the publishers or printers would be liable in any manner to any person by reason of any mistake or omission in this publication or for any action taken or omitted to be taken or advice rendered or accepted on the basis of this work. For any defect in printing or binding the publishers will be liable only to replace the defective copy by another copy of this work then available.

Contents

List of Tables

Foreword

राष्ट्रीय प्राकृतिक चिकित्सा संस्थान
आयुष मंत्रालय, भारत सरकार
'बापू भवन', मातोश्री रमाबाई अंबेडकर रोड,
पुणे 411 001
दूरभाष : 020-26059682 / 3 / 4 / 5 फैक्स : 020-26059131
ई-मेल : ninpune@bharatmail.co.in
वेबसाईट : ninpune.ayush.gov.in

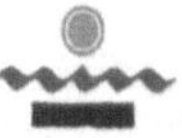

NATIONAL INSTITUTE OF NATUROPATHY
Ministry of Ayush, Govt. of India
'Bapu Bhavan', Matoshree Ramabai Ambedkar Road,
Pune 411 001
Phone: 020-26059682 / 3 / 4 / 5 Fax : 020-26059131
Email : ninpune@bharatmail.co.in
Website : ninpune.ayush.gov.in

Indians have long understood that life revolves around water, recognizing its fundamental role in sustaining life and promoting health. The importance of water in Indian culture and medicine is evident in the ancient texts, which describe numerous modalities of using water for therapeutic purposes, including baths, compresses, and steam treatments. From ancient Roman baths to contemporary spa treatments, the principles of hydrotherapy have evolved, refined, and stood the test of time, proving their efficacy and significance in the holistic approach to health and wellness.

In this "Handbook of Hydrotherapy," we draw upon the profound wisdom and extensive research presented in the seminal work "Rational Hydrotherapy" by J.H. Kellogg. Dr. Kellogg's contributions to the field of hydrotherapy are monumental. His systematic approach and scientific rigor have provided a solid foundation upon which modern hydrotherapy practices are built. Through his pioneering work, Dr. Kellogg illuminated the therapeutic potentials of water, emphasizing its role in promoting health, preventing illness, and aiding recovery.

This handbook aims to distil the core principles and practical applications from Dr. Kellogg's comprehensive treatise. It seeks to make the profound benefits of hydrotherapy accessible to both practitioners and enthusiasts alike. By presenting the essential techniques and therapies in a concise and practical format, this book serves as an invaluable resource for those looking to integrate hydrotherapy into their health regimen or professional practice.

It is clear that this "Handbook of Hydrotherapy" will inspire and empower the readers, Naturopathy Enthusiast and physicians to embrace the principles of hydrotherapy, enriching the understanding and practice of this remarkable natural therapy. Let the wisdom of Dr. J.H. Kellogg guide you on a journey towards greater health and vitality.

Prof. (Dr.) K Satya Lakshmi,
Director

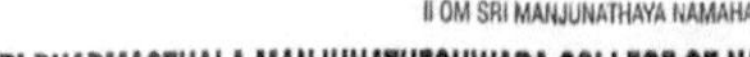

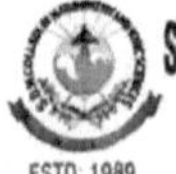

II OM SRI MANJUNATHAYA NAMAHA II

SRI DHARMASTHALA MANJUNATHESHWARA COLLEGE OF NATUROPATHY AND YOGIC SCIENCES

Affiliated to Rajiv Gandhi University of Health Sciences and Recognized by Govt. of Karnataka
Managed by: S. D. M. Educational Society (Regd.), Ujire
President: DR. D. VEERENDRA HEGGADE

ESTD: 1989

CENTRE FOR EXCELLENCE IN CLINICAL RESEARCH BY MINISTRY OF AYUSH, GOVERNMENT OF INDIA

Dr. PRASHANTH SHETTY
PRINCIPAL

Ref: SDMCNYS/

Dr. Vrinda Bedekar, an esteemed alumna of our SDM College of Naturopathy & Yogic Sciences, Ujire, has always stood out as a remarkable student. From her early days, she exhibited a keen interest in writing and a deep contemplation of nature, often immersing herself in her thoughts and studies.

It is with great pleasure that I write this foreword for her book, "Handbook of Hydrotherapy." This book serves as a comprehensive and quick reference for all BNYS students, compiling and presenting the seminal works of renowned hydrotherapists from the past. Dr. Vrinda has adeptly highlighted the psychological, physiological, biochemical, and autonomic neurological effects of water applications in a simple and engaging manner, making the content easy to understand and retain.

In-depth knowledge of these multifaceted effects of water treatments is crucial, as hydrotherapy is a fundamental component of nature cure treatments. Through this book, the historical practices of hydrotherapy can be well comprehended and effectively applied in contemporary therapeutic practices.

My best wishes to Dr. Vrinda for her commendable contribution to the field of naturopathy through this book. Her extensive research and numerous references to authoritative sources enhance the credibility and richness of the content. Upon reviewing the book, I believe it has the potential to be transformed from a handbook into a comprehensive textbook.

Furthermore, I am confident that this book will inspire our faculty and Deans to write more books on naturopathy and yoga, thereby enriching the academic resources available to students and practitioners alike.

Dr.Prashanth Shetty
PRINCIPAL
Recipient Karnataka Rajyotsava award 2023
BNYS, M.Sc, PhD
Principal
Sri D.M. College of
Naturopathy & Yogic Science

P.O. UJIRE - 674240(D. Kannada) — College offering BNYS and M.D. Programs in Naturopathy and Yogic Sciences
UJIRE 574 240, DAKSHINA KANNADA, KARNATAKA, INDIA
Ph.: (08256) 236188, 236343, +91-9448252696 FAX: (08256) 236844 Email: sdmcnys@gmail.com website: www.sdmbnys.in

Preface

Hydrotherapy is an integral part of Nature cure treatments. Various forms of water treatments when systematically employed with a sound knowledge provide wonderful therapeutic benefits. This is evident by the works of many hydrotherapy practitioners all over the world. J.H. Kellogg, Winternitz, Currie, Fleury, Sebastian Kniepp and many more to mention whose work provide a firm foundation for therapeutic effects of water. In spite of various books on Hydrotherapy Dr. J. H.Kellogg's "Rational Hydrotherapy" remains as an encyclopedia for all Nature Cure practitioners & Students.

Gathering the basics of hydrotherapy in a concise handy book is the main idea of writing this book. 'Hand Book of Hydrotherapy' is the work mainly from Kellogg's voluminous work of "Rational Hydrotherapy" This is done to help the students to understand the physiological effects of water in a better way. It can be a quick guide for the students. In the light of this knowledge strong scientific evidence can be established by the practitioners of hydrotherapy.

– Dr. Vrinda Bedekar
BNYS, MS (Counselling & Psychotherapy),
MD (Clinical Yoga)

Acknowledgement

I express my deep sense of gratitude to:

My teachers of SDM College of Naturopathy & Yogic Sciences, Ujire.

Prof.(Dr.) K. Satya Lakshmi, Director, National Institute of Naturopathy, Pune who was generous enough to write the foreward.

Dr. Prashanth Shetty, Prinicipal, SDM College of Naturopathy& Yogic Sciences, Ujire for going through the content and providing valuable inputs & writing a foreword.

The management of Alva's College of Naturopathy & Yogic Sciences, Moodabidri for wonderful teaching & clinical experience during my service in the Institution.

Dr. Vanitha S Shetty, Principal and colleagues of Alva's College of Naturopathy & Yogic Sciences, Moodbidri for invaluable support during my service.

Dr. Vidyarani, Wellness Specialist, Yo 1 Health Resort, New York, for her unconditional love and support.

Dr. Prashanth B.K, Principal, Colleagues & Management of Prasanna College of Ayurveda & Hospital for the continuous support & providing a beautiful working atmosphere.

Dr. M.S Krishnamurthy, Professor & HOD, Dept. of Rasa Shastra & Bhaishajya Kalpana, Alva's Ayurveda Medical College and Hospital, Moodbidri for his guidance to publish this book through Notion Press.

Dr. S.B.Hegde MD, FRCP, Cardiac Physician, Hegde Health Complex, Shimoga, a mentor & a constant source of encouragement at all times.

My dear students who are the constant inspiration for teaching & book writing work.

My Parents, Husband, Children, In laws & family members for the unconditional love & support during my professional journey.

Introduction

Water is a unique substance and it is the key constituent of all living organisms. Its universal availability has made it as an agent to prevent and cure diseases since time immemorial. It was around the water that many ancient civilizations were born. Water was regarded as a holy substance which can act as a purifier and wash away the sins of people. Plunging into the holy water of Niles, Jordan and Ganges by Egyptians, Israelites and Hindus respectively was the ancient practice to heal the body and soul. Such was an intimate connection of human being with water. History of use of water for curing diseases is evident by different nations all over the world. Egyptians, Greeks, Hindus, Romans, Hebrews, Chinese all included water as a remedial agent during different diseases.

The term 'Hydrotherapy' is derived from the Greek word 'Hydro' means water and 'Therapia' means healing. That is healing of the diseases through water. In a broader sense Hydrotherapy is the methodical application of water on the body either internally or externally in its various forms and temperatures for the prevention and treatment of diseases.

Structure & Function of Skin in Relation to Hydrotherapy

Skin is the largest organ of the body contributes one sixth of the body weight. It covers 20 square feet area in an adult. It covers the underlying structures & is the first line of defence against microorganisms.

Skin is divided into 3 main layers:

1. Epidermis

2. Dermis

3. Hypodermis or Subcutaneous layer

1. **Epidermis:** This is the outermost layer of the skin & has an average thickness of 0.1mm& it is avascular. This layer of skin consists of keratinized, stratified squamous epithelium. Depending on its location in the body skin consists of 4 or 5 layers of epithelial cells. Skin with four layers of cells is called as thin skin & that with five layers is called as thick skin. Skin overlying the palms & sole is thick skin & all the other parts of the body are

covered with thin skin. Skin over the eyelid is the thinnest.

2. The epidermal layer is replaced every 3to 4 weeks by shedding off. There are 4 specialised cells in the epidermal layer. Keratinocytes • Melanocytes • Merkel Cells • Langerhan Cells (immune function).

3. **Dermis:** Dermis is present immediately below the epidermis. It contains nerves, blood & lymph vessels, hair follicles & sweat glands. It gives strength, shape, smoothness & elasticity to the skin. It is composed of two layers: Superficial papillary layer & deep reticular layer.

    a. **Papillary layer:** The finger like projections into the lower layer of the epidermis forms the papillae & hence the name. This layer consists of fibroblasts, few adipocytes, numerous small blood vessels, lymphatic capillaries, nerve fibres, phagocytes, defensive cells & nerve endings sensitive to touch, cold, heat, pain & pressure.

    b. **Reticular layer:** Tight meshwork of fibres in this layer produces net like (reticulated) appearance & hence its name. This layer is highly vascularized with abundant supply of sensory & sympathetic nerves. Elastin (yellow) fibres present in this layer provides elasticity to the skin. Collagen (white) fibres provide shape & tensile strength to the skin. Water binding property of collagen keeps the skin hydrated.

3. **Hypodermis or Subcutaneous layer (superficial fascia):** Hypodermis is a layer below the dermis and connects the skin to the underlying fascia of bones & muscles. This layer consists of well vascularized loose areolar tissue & adipose tissue. It stores fat, provides cushioning effect to underlying structures & serves as an insulator by preventing loss of heat from the skin.

Accessory structures of the skin: Hair, nails, sweat glands & sebaceous glands are accessory structures of the skin.

Hair: Hair originates deep in the dermis travels through the epidermis & projects out of the skin through an opening. The external hair is made of keratin & it is dead. We do not have sensation on external hair. Each hair root is connected with a smooth muscle called erector pili. This muscle contracts in response to signals from sympathetic nervous system making the external hair to stand up producing goose bumps.

Sweat glands: There are two types of sweat glands – **Eccrine & Apocrine glands**.

Eccrine sweat glands produce hypotonic sweat for temperature regulation. Human beings have 2-4 million eccrine sweat glands. They are found on both hairy &

non hairy parts of the body with the denser distribution on the palms & soles. They start functioning at 2 to 3 years of age & the number of glands remain fixed throughout the life.

Apocrine sweat glands: These are found on the hairy parts of the body (armpits, genitals) and are attached to the hair follicle. Apocrine glands are larger than the eccrine sweat glands. They lie deeper in the dermis sometimes reaching to hypodermis. Apocrine sweat is subjected to bacterial decomposition & is the cause of body odour.

Sebaceous glands: These glands produce sebum on the skin surface which is a mixture of lipids. Sebum helps to lubricate the skin & hairs. These glands are found all over the body except on the palms & soles. Sebum secretion is stimulated by hormones which are active only after puberty.

Composition of sweat: Sweat is secreted through 2.6 million skin pores. 30% of the body waste is excreted through sweating. The composition of sweat is different from eccrine & apocrine glands. Eccrine sweat consist of water, minerals (sodium, potassium, magnesium & calcium) metabolic end products (lactate, ammonia & urea) & unmetabolized pharmaceutical drugs. Apocrine sweat is basically oily & odourless secretion. Along with the identical mineral & metabolites they also contain protein, lipids & steroids.

Regulation of sweating: An increased body temperature is perceived by the central & skin thermoreceptors. Preoptic area of hypothalamus consists of heat sensitive & cold sensitive neurons. This information is processed by preoptic area of hypothalamus and sets up sweating mechanism. Nerve impulses are transmitted from hypothalamus to the spinal cord through autonomic nerves and from there through sympathetic nerves to the skin over the body. Sweat glands are supplied by cholinergic (secrete acetylcholine) nerve fibres. Epinephrine & nor epinephrine in the blood secreted after the exercise can stimulate sweat glands to lose the excess heat.

Note: Whole body sweating rate is the product of density of active sweat glands and rate of secretion per gland.

Functions of the skin: Skin has wide variety of functions:

1. Protection

2. Temperature regulation

3. Sensory function

4. Synthesis of Vit. D

1. **Protection:** Skin protects the body from wind, water, UV light, harmful chemicals & various microorganisms. It prevents water loss.

2. **Temperature regulation:** Skin is associated with sympathetic nervous system in regulating the internal temperature. Through the insensible & sensible perspiration body tries to cool itself. Sweat secreted through the insensible perspiration is about 500 ml/day. High external temperature or vigorous exercise increases the body temperature. This stimulates the sweat glands through the sympathetic nervous system to produce large amount of sweat. About 0.7 to 1.5 L of sweat is produced per hour in an active person. Evaporation of sweat cools the body through heat dissipation. When the body is exposed to excess heat or cold following mechanism sets in to regulate the temperature.

When the body is warm:

- **Vasodilatation of skin vessels:** Arterioles in the dermis dilate to carry large volume of blood to the skin surface so that heat is dissipated. This is due to the inhibition of sympathetic centres in posterior hypothalamus which cause vasoconstriction. This causes redness of the skin as seen in vigorous activity.

- **Stimulation of sweating:** Every 1°C increase in the body temperature removes 10 times the basal rate of heat production through excess sweating.

- **Reduced heat production:** Through the inhibition of shivering & chemical thermogenesis heat production is reduced.

When the body is cool:

- **Vasoconstriction of skin vessels:** Arterioles in the dermis constrict to reduce the heat loss by restricting the blood flow. This is prominent in the tip of the nose & in the tips of the digits. This is due to the stimulation of sympathetic centres in the posterior hypothalamus.

- **Piloerection:** Contraction of the erector pili muscle attached to the hair follicles causes straightening of cutaneous hair. This is mediated through sympathetic stimulation.

- **Increased heat production:** Through the stimulation of shivering & chemical thermogenesis heat production is increased.

- Marked reduction of skin temperature can lead to freezing of the skin (frostbite) to preserve the core heat.

3. **Sensory function:** The rich innervations of the skin helps us to sense the environment and respond accordingly. Sensory cutaneous receptors are present in the epidermis & dermis which are the part of somato sensory system. Skin sensory receptors are broadly named

as mechanoreceptors (Ruffini, Meissner and Pacinian corpuscles, Merkel disk and free nerve endings), thermoreceptors and nociceptors.

4. **Synthesis of Vit. D**: Vit D is synthesized in the epidermis when exposed to Sunlight. Along with its role in bone & teeth mineralization it provides immunity against various microbial infections.

Nerve supply of the skin: Skin is a highly sensitive organ densely supplied with different types of nerves.

Skin is supplied by both somatic & autonomic (mainly sympathetic but in face also parasympathetic) nervous system. Somatic sensory nerves mediate pain, temperature, proprioception, vibration, light touch, pressure sensation to the central nervous system. There are special receptors & nerve endings to mediate these sensation. Different sensory nerve fibres innervate these receptors. They are Aβ, Aδ & C fibres classified according to the diameter & speed of the impulse.

Autonomic nerve fibres in the skin innervate sweat glands, sebaceous glands, arector pilori muscle, blood vessels, lymphatic vessels, arteriovenous anastomoses & hair follicles. It maintains cutaneous homeostasis by regulating vasomotor, pilomotor activities & glandular secretions.

Skin receptors:

- **Light touch:** Meissner's corpuscles, Merkel cells. These receptors are located in the skin of the palms, soles, lips, eyelids, external genitals and nipples.

- **Vibration & deep pressure:** Pacinian corpuscles. Every square centimetre contains 14 pressure receptors.

- **Deep Pressure & stretching of skin:** Ruffini end organs

- **Pain:** Nociceptors. They are numerous & each centimetre of skin contains about 200 pain receptors.

- **Thermoreceptors:** skin registers both cold & warmth. Thermoreceptors are distributed throughout the body. They are denser in the face & ears. Ears & nose feel colder than the rest of the body in winter season for this reason. Cold receptors are more than the hot receptors. Each square centimetre of skin contains 6 cold receptors & one hot receptor.

Sensation	Mediating Nerve fibre
Touch	Aβ fibres
Touch & pressure	Aβ fibres (Merkel disk and Ruffini corpuscles), Aδ fibres (free nerve endings)
Vibration	Aβ fibres
Temperature	Aδ fibres (cold receptors) C fibres (warmth receptors)
Pain	Aδ fibres (cold receptors) C fibres (warmth receptors)

Table 1: Different nerve fibres conducting skin sensations

S. No	Point of stimulation	Cold receptors	Hot receptors
1.	Start perceiving the temperature	<95 °F	> 86 °F
2.	Maximum	77°F	113°F
3.	No stimulation	<41°F	>113°F

Table 2: Thermoreceptor response at various temperatures

Note:

- Cold receptors are not stimulated below 41°F. This is the reason why feet & hands become numb when submerged in ice water.

- Hot receptors are not stimulated beyond 113°F, pain receptors are activated at this stage to avoid damage to the skin & underlying tissues.

- Deep temperature receptors are found in the spinal cord, abdominal organs and in or around the large veins in the thorax & upper abdomen. They sense the changes in the core temperature.

- Human body temperature changes by 1°C for every 25° to 30° C changes in the external temperature.

- Tactile sensitivity: Tactile pressure sensitivity varies in different parts of the body. It is highest on the face followed by trunk, upper limbs (arms & fingers) & then the lower limbs (thighs, calf & feet).

03

Nervous System in Relation to Hydrotherapy

Vasomotor Centre: This centre is situated bilaterally in the reticular substance of the medulla and in the lower third of the Pons. There are three important areas in this centre, they are:

1. **Vasoconstrictor area:** present bilaterally in the anterolateral part of the upper medulla. The neurons from this area reach at all levels of spinal cord.

2. **Vasodilator area:** Present bilaterally in the anterolateral part of the lower half of the medulla. The fibers from these neurons inhibit the action of the vasoconstrictor area and produce vasodilatation.

3. **Sensory area:** Present bilaterally in the posterolateral portions of the medulla and lower pons. This area receives sensory inputs from the circulatory system. Output signals from this area regulate the activities of the vasoconstrictor and vasodilator areas of the vasomotor center.

Autonomic Nervous System & Circulation:

Body circulation is mainly controlled by Sympathetic Nervous System & partially by Parasympathetic nervous system. Through the thoracic & first one or two lumbar spinal nerves sympathetic vasomotor fibers exit the spinal cord. They pass into the sympathetic chain on either side of the vertebral column and run through the different routes to innervate the vessels of the internal organs & peripheral vessels.

Sympathetic innervation is seen in almost all the arteries, arterioles & veins, except in the capillaries. Sympathetic stimulation constricts the vessels & increases the activity of the heart through the increased heart rate & force of contraction. Parasympathetic stimulation has a major influence in controlling the heart rate through the vagus nerve. As a result there is decrease in heart rate & its force of contraction.

Vasomotor Tone: Normally blood vessels in the body maintain a partial state of contraction due to the continuous signals sent by the vasoconstrictor area of the vasomotor centre. This is called as vasomotor tone.

Norepinephrine: Norepinephrine is the substance secreted by the vasoconstrictor nerves. This acts on the vascular smooth muscles to causes vasoconstriction.

Adrenal medulla & sympathetic vasoconstriction:
Sympathetic signals are distributed to the blood vessels & to the adrenal medulla simultaneously. On stimulation

adrenal medulla secretes epinephrine & norepinephrine in to the circulation. They are distributed to the whole body & directly act on the blood vessels to cause vasoconstriction. In some tissues epinephrine causes vasodilatation.

04

Properties of Water

Therapeutic effects of water are due to its three unique properties. They are

1. Property of absorbing & communicating Heat
2. Ability to dissolve substances
3. Change of state property

1. Property of Absorbing & Communicating Heat:

Water has a high specific heat capacity when compared to other substances. Due to this, it takes up more time to heat and an equal amount of time to lose its heat. Therefore the temperature of water rises and drops gradually when compared with other substances hence it is used as a potent therapeutic agent in Hydrotherapy. This property is essential to regulate environmental temperature.

Note: Heat is the amount of thermal energy. Temperature is the measure of kinetic energy of a substance.

Specific Heat Capacity: It is the amount of heat required to raise the temperature of one gram of a substance by one degree Celsius. Specific Heat Capacity of water is: 4182 J/kg°C. With the high specific heat capacity water can regulate internal body temperature. This property has lot of advantages when we use water as a therapeutic agent. It can absorb heat and communicate heat to the body when applied at different temperatures. For eg: Fomentation, hot compresses etc. Water remains hot for a longer duration and also enhances vasodilatation and movement of blood through the area. Application of a cold compress over the forehead during fever absorbs heat from the body and tries to reduce the temperature.

Note: Since water has high specific heat capacity it heats up & cools down slowly.

2. Ability to dissolve substances/ Solvent property:

Water is known as universal solvent. It can dissolve many substances including simple salts, smaller molecules like sugar & metabolites, larger molecules like nucleic acid & proteins. Because of this property transport of essential molecules takes place through the blood stream. For eg transport of Glucose, oxygen, sodium chloride, amino acids etc. These substances are called as hydrophilic (water loving) substances.

Carbonic acid gas, Urea, bilirubin are some of the metabolic products which are excreted out from the body through different systems because of their solubility in water. Therefore water is utilized as a cleansing agent both externally and internally.

Internal use of water can be in the form of water drinking, enema, gastric lavage, colon hydrotherapy etc. molecules, ranging from simple salts through small molecules such as sugars and metabolites to very large molecules such as proteins and nucleic acids. In fact water is sometimes called the universal solven can dissolve a remarkable variety of important molecules, ranging from simple salts through small molecules such as sugars and metabolites to very large molecules such as proteins and nucleic acids. In fact water is sometimes called the universal olven

3. Change of State: water has the ability to change into liquid, solid and gaseous states.ie as water, ice and vapour. It can be used for treatment in all three different states.Liquid state of water is used at different temperatures ranging from cold 32°F to very hot 104°F.

Ice and vapor can be used at extremes of temperatures to produce analgesia and decongestion.

Water in its liquid state is used as Baths, Compresses, Packs, Douches and Irrigations. At solid state it is used as packs or compresses, at gaseous state it is used in vapor baths.

CLASSIFICATION OF WATER TEMPERATURE FOR THERAPUTIC APPLICATIONS

S. NO	TEMPERTATURE	°F	°C
1.	VERY COLD	32 - 55	-1 - 13
2.	COLD	55 - 65	13 - 18
3.	COOL	65 - 80	18 - 27
4.	TEPID	80 - 92	27 - 33
5.	WARM (NEUTRAL)	92 - 98 (92 - 95)	33 - 37 (33 TO 35)
6.	HOT	98 - 104	37 - 40
7.	VERY HOT	104 & ABOVE	40 & ABOVE

Table 3: Classification of Water Temperature

05

Physiological Effects of Water

When water comes in contact with the body (internally or externally) it produces certain physiological effects. These effects are attributed to water's unique qualities as a:

1. Nutrient: water acts as a nutrient which enters into the every cell & acts a mediator to supply nutrients & remove waste from the tissues.

2. Abstractor of heat: It removes excess heat from the body by contact & evaporation.

3. Communicator of heat: It communicates heat to the body.

4. Agent that produces mechanical or percutient effects.

The physiological changes that follow the application of water are of three types:

1. Action or Primary Effect (includes Circulatory action & thermic action)

2. Reaction or secondary Effect (includes Circulatory reaction & thermic reaction)

3. Remote Effect

1. **Action or Primary Effect:** The immediate effects that accompany hot or cold application are called as primary effect or action.

2. **Reaction or secondary Effect:** Series of vital processes which follow hot or cold application are called as secondary effect or reaction.

3. **Remote effect:** Effect of series of applications which modify the normal or pathological nutritive processes are called as remote effects.

Reaction, its types & variations:

Reaction is mainly of two types i.e. Circulatory reaction & Thermic reaction

1. **Circulatory reaction:** Changes that are observed in the blood circulation due to the constriction or dilatation of blood vessels brought by hot or cold applications.

2. **Thermic reaction:** Effort of the body to restore the equilibrium of the body temperature following hot or cold application.

Thermic reaction following a general cold application:

Fleury, Liebermeister, Bottey and others have proved that general cold application to the skin or mucous membrane lower the surface temperature and internal temperature of the body.

In most of the cases there will be a slight initial rise of temperature before the actual reduction of internal temperature. This initial rise of temperature starts with cold application and progresses for about 10 to 12 minutes afterwards. This is followed by steady decline and temperature reaches to normal.

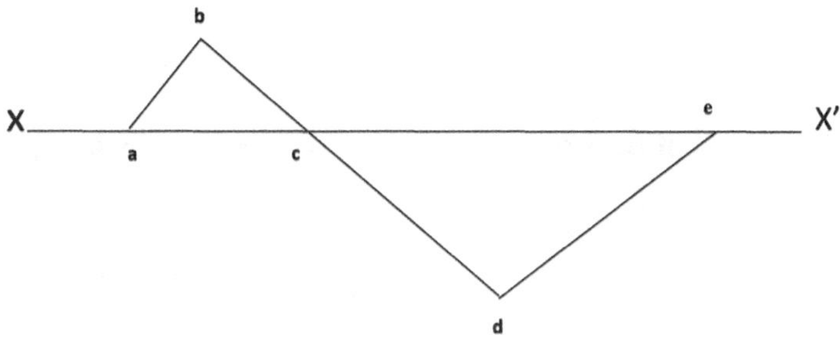

Fig 1: Vital movements with general cold application

xx' – Normal temperature

ab – slight rise in internal temperature

bcd – fall in the internal temperature

de – Reaction

abcd – Action

Modification of thermic reaction:

Under different conditions thermic reaction to cold will be modified.

For eg: Initial increase of temperature can be further increased with the heavy exercise or hot bath before the cold application.

Initial increase of temperature is absent with Warm or tepid application. (80 - 92°F)

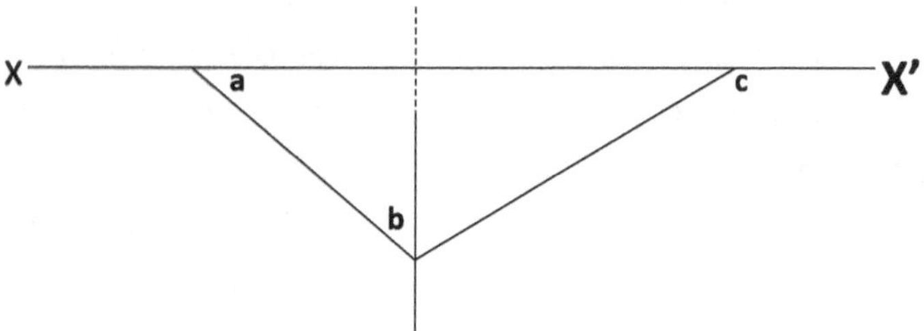

Fig 2: Vital movements with warm or tepid bath

xx' – Normal temperature

ab – Action (cooling of the body)

bc – Reaction

Vertical dotted line shows the point of separation between action and reaction.

Variations in reaction according to the vitality of the subject under treatment:

1. Second Reaction

2. Incomplete Reaction

3. Oscillatory Reaction

1. **Second Reaction:** If a reaction is set in after an application is made and a renewed application will bring about another reaction with a lesser intensity. This is called as second reaction. In a feeble and fatigued subject secondary reaction may not occur.

In a healthy and vigorous subjects with the successive applications third or fourth reaction can occur but with the lesser intensity.

2. **Incomplete Reaction:** Absence of prompt reaction following an application is called as incomplete reaction. Due to this the subject experiences unpleasant symptoms like giddiness, prolonged chills, weakness, nausea, fainting etc.

3. **Oscillatory Reaction:** Following a cold bath succeeding reactions become weaker than the previous one. This is called oscillatory reaction. This is observed occasionally. Blood rapidly rushes towards the skin during first reaction & it is quickly cooled by evaporation. Following reduced skin temperature produces weaker reaction in the next attempt.

Manipulation of reaction in different clinical conditions to produce the desired effect:

1. Suppression of reaction: Reaction has to be suppressed in local or general applications to produce the sedative effects.

General applications where reaction is suppressed:

- Prolonged tepid bath for fever
- Prolonged neutral bath for insomnia

Local applications where reaction is suppressed:

Prolonged application of cold to arrest local inflammation as in cases of congestive headache, pain, hemorrhage etc.

Note: Reaction can be enhanced with friction, strong pressure or by protecting evaporation during the application.eg:

- Cold immersion with the friction to reduce fever
- Short cold douche for tonic effect
- Heating compress to a rheumatic joint protected by evaporation.

TONIC & ATONIC REACTION

S. NO	EFFECT ON	TONIC REACTION	ATONIC REACTION
1.	**Skin Vessels**	Vasodilatation	Vasoconstriction
2.	**Color of the skin**	Red	Pale
3.	**Pulse Rate**	Reduced	Increased
4.	**Arterial Tension**	Increased	Reduced
5.	**Skin action**	Increased	Decreased
6.	**Temperature**	Reduced	Reduced
7.	**Sensation**	Energetic	Tiredness
8.	**Muscle capacity**	Increased	Decreased

9.	**Amount of Respired air**	Increased	Decreased
10.	**Heat production**	Increased	Decreased

Table 4: Tonic & Atomic reaction

Tonic Reaction: The reaction following cold application is excitant or tonic in character. Therefore this is termed as tonic reaction.

Atonic Reaction: The reaction following hot application are depressant or atonic in character. Therefore this is termed as atonic reaction.

Conditions that control reaction:

Method of water application (percutient or non percutient application)

1. Temperature of water application

2. Duration of application

3. Condition of the patient:

    a. Febrile or non febrile

    b. Weak or strong

    c. Fat or thin

    d. Relaxed or tiered

    e. Skin warm or cool

4. Capacity to produce heat

5. Capacity to recuperate the heat loss & supporting the heat loss without any problem to vital organs.

6. Condition of the nervous system during application

7. Capacity to adapt to the cold application

8. Mental state of the patient (nervous, anxious, cheerful etc)

Major types of effects of water application:

Schuller's experiments concluded that application of

- Cold water to a nerve trunk caused contraction of the cerebral vessels.

- Warm water to a nerve trunk caused dilatation of the cerebral vessels.

General applications to the skin in the form of compresses and baths produced reverse effects i.e.

- Warm bath caused dilatation of the surface vessels and contraction in the cerebral vessels.

- Cold bath caused contraction of the surface vessels and dilatation of the cerebral vessels.

These observations are suggestive of two types of effects during the application of water on the surface. They are:

1. Reflex effect

2. Mechanical or Derivative effect

In all types of applications both of the above effects are produced. But in local applications reflex effect is more pronounced as the area involved is smaller. In general applications mechanical effect is more prominent. The reflex effect seen in general applications is immediately followed by mechanical effect due to the internal movement of the blood from the periphery.

This movement of blood from the superficial vessels to the interior of the body is called as **retrostasis.** Cold application to a large skin surface produces marked retrostasis.

SUMMARY OF PRIMARY & SECONDARY EFFECTS OF SHORT COLD APPLICATION

S. NO	EFFECT	ACTION	REACTION
1.	**SKIN** **a. Blood vessels**	Superficial V.C (in small vessels) Internal V.D after a brief contraction.	Superficial V.D, Internal V.C
	b. Color	Pallor	Redness
	c. Texture	Gooseflesh appearance & roughness	Soft, smooth & supple

	d. Sensation	Chillness Trembling, shivering, chattering of teeth, Painful & distressing sensation of constriction	Warmth Comfort & well being
	e. Temperature	Cooling	Heating
2.	**PULSE**	Initial Quickening then slowing, increased tension	Slowing, increased tension
3.	**RESPIRATION**	Initially checked then quick deep gasping	Free, slower & deeper
4.	**INTERNAL TEMPERATURE**	Slightly increased	Reduced
5.	**PERSPIRATION**	Checked	Increased

Table 5: Primary & Secondary Effects of Short Cold Application

SUMMARY OF PRIMARY & SECONDARY EFFECTS OF INTENSE SHORT GENERAL HOT APPLICATION

S. NO.	EFFECT	ACTION	REACTION
1.	**SKIN** **a. Blood Vessels**	Brief contraction later surface V.D (in small vessels)	V.C

	b. Color	Initial pallor following prior redness, later dusky redness	Pallor
	c. Texture	Goose flesh appearance, mild shivering	Smooth, soft & moist
	d. Temperature	Heating	Gradual cooling
2.	**PULSE**	Slowed, later quickened, increased tension	Regular, decreased tension
3.	**RESPIRATION**	Checked initially, later frequent, CO_2 reduced	Regular, superficial & free
4.	**INTERNAL TEMPERATURE**	Increased due to reduced heat elimination	Reduced due to increased heat elimination & reduced heat production
5.	**PERSPIRATION**	First checked later increased	Reduced
6.	**NERVOUS SYSTEM**	General excitation (moderate temp.) sensation of comfort & relief	Sedation, sense of depression & drowsiness
7.	**MUSCLES**	Excitation	Weakness

Table 6: Primary & Secondary Effects of Intense Short General Hot Application

PHYSIOLOGICAL EFFECTS OF COLD APPLICATIONS:

Means of cold applications: ice, cold water, cold air, by the evaporation of water or volatile liquids from the surface of the body.

General effects:

- ✓ Cold is primary depressant or sedative. i.e. application of cold lessens the vital activities and lowers the body temperature in the action phase.

- ✓ It is Secondary excitant i.e. application of cold increases vital activities and restores the body temperature back to normal in the reaction phase. These changes are brought by the reaction of the body against the sedative influence of cold application.

1. In Short cold applications reaction follows immediately. The intensity of reaction depends upon the temperature and the mode of application.

   For eg: short cold applications in the form of a shower causes contraction of the blood vessels in the skin and the internal organs. Since the application is for a shorter duration reaction sets in quickly by causing active dilatation of the blood vessels internally followed by externally.

2. A prolonged moderate cold application (65°-80° F) causes prolonged contraction of the superficial vessels and reflexly related internal vessels.

Primary effect of cold	Depressant/ sedative
Secondary effect of cold	Excitant / Stimulant
Short cold application	Sudden contraction of skin & reflex internal vessels Followed by dilatation of reflex internal & skin vessels
Prolonged moderate cold application	Prolonged contraction of skin & reflex internal vessels

Table 7: Summary of effect of cold

Conditions that influence reaction in cold applications:

The degree and intensity of reaction in cold treatments can be enhanced by adapting certain measures before, during and after the application.

Measures given before the cold application

- Wrapping the subject with warm cloths
- Exposure to a warm room
- Hot bath
- Drinking hot water or hot drinks
- Exercise according to the strength of the subject
- Hot enema
- Friction to the skin until warm or red

Note: Intense reaction will be observed if the subject is healthy and one with the warm, dry or slightly moist skin.

Measures given during the cold application

- Lower temperature of the bath
- Short and sudden application
- Addition of pressure with Application
- Friction during the bath
- Alternate or revulsive spray or douche with the greater temperature difference.

Measures taken after the cold application

- Exposure to warm room
- Wearing warm clothing
- Hot water drinking
- Exercise according to the strength of the patient
- Friction of the body surface by self or attendant (with the hand, rough towel)

Conditions that discourage reaction in general cold applications:

- Elderly people
- Infants
- Exhaustion due to excess exercise, loss of sleep or due to nervous exhaustion.

- Obesity

- Rheumatic Diathesis

- Impaired skin functioning

- Profuse sweating with exhaustion

- Severe nervous agitation

- Very cold skin

- Chills before or immediately after the application

- Dislike towards cold applications.

EFFECTS OF COLD UPON SKIN:

1. Contraction of the small blood vessels
2. Reduction or suspension of sweating
3. Reduced heat elimination & Enhanced heat production.
4. Reduced tactile sensation

1. Contraction of the small blood vessels:

Primary effect/ action phase of cold:

➢ Cold or very cold (32° to 65°F) applications for short duration produces pale &cold skin. Pallor of the skin is seen initially due to the spasm of the small arteries, veins & capillaries.

➢ When the same application is continued the surface becomes blue, the physiological changes in the action phase are as follows:

- Exhaustion & relaxation of the muscles of the small veins.

- Muscles of arterioles are in active contracted state

- Capillaries are contracted

- Pressure in the veins reduced therefore blood flow slows down.

- Formation of reduced haemoglobin in the venules which are distended with the blood.

- The skin looks blue or purple in colour.

Secondary effect/ Reaction phase of cold:

When the application is withdrawn without prolonging it the surface colour changes from pale or blue to redness as a result of active dilatation of the smaller arteries in the skin.

Note: Smaller vessels show the same effect as that of cold water application with Percussion, slapping & friction movements i.e initial stimulation of vasoconstrictors followed by vasodilatation.

2. Reduction or suspension of sweating:

Action Phase:

- ✓ General cold applications initially diminish the activity of sweat glands and then increase it. Experiments of Kellogg reveal that the action of cold is quicker when compared to the action of hot to excite the sweat glands.

Suspending the activity of the sweat glands of the entire skin can also be brought by the application of cold to a very smaller area through the reflex effect.eg: feet, shoulders, hands etc.

Abrupt suspension of perspiration is contraindicated in fatigue and in sweating stage of malaria.

Reaction Phase:

✓ In the reaction phase sweat gland activity is restarted and enhanced considerably.

3. Reduced heat elimination & Enhanced heat production.

Action Phase:

Contraction of blood vessels brought about by the application of cold results in reduced blood flow through the skin vessels. This greatly reduces heat elimination from the body. There is simultaneous increase in the heat production as a reflex effect.

Reaction Phase:

Active dilatation of the blood vessels enhances the skin circulation. Large volume of blood is exposed to the cooling effect of atmospheric air. This results in increased heat elimination.

Prolonged cold:

With the prolonged cold application temperature of the skin & underlying muscles is reduced. So this stops heat production in the muscles.

4. Reduced tactile sensation:

Tactile sensation is at its maximum near the body temperature. Temperature below 92° to 98° F reduces the intensity of touch sensation. Applications lower than 32°F do not stimulate temperature receptors; they excite the pain receptors & give rise to pain.

Applications that reduce the tactile sensibility are:

- Short application of ice or very cold water
- Prolonged application of cold water

Note:

1. Gradual & sudden application of cold water initially brings different sensations. Gradual exposure to cold is more painful than the sudden exposure. In sudden applications sensation is generalised when compared to the gradual application where the sensation is concentrated to a smaller area. So each exposure excites the receptors in the smaller areas.

2. A fine spray & a douche at the same temperature gives different sensation. It senses as fine spray

is cooler than the douche. The strong mechanical effect of douche stuns the skin. Thus it lessens the skin sensibility.

For the same reason cold immersion bath produces more shock than the douche at the same temperature.

EFFECT OF COLD ON MUCOUS MEMBRANE

- ✓ Due to the smaller number of sensory nerve fibres mucous membrane is less sensitive to the thermic impressions made on it. Otherwise the effect of cold is same as that of the skin. As the mucous membrane is richly supplied with vasomotor and sympathetic fibres the desired reflex effects will be produced.

- ✓ A required quantity of water taken in to the stomach produces noticeable effects than external application of water on the equal area. Drinking cold water (Internal application) can reduce the body temperature and pulse rate.

EFFECTS OF COLD UPON CIRCULATION:

Action Phase:

General Cold applications quicken the heart beat and increase the arterial tension. The initial quickening of heart beat is due to the shock experienced by the sudden cold applications. Cold applied to the skin reflexley influences the nervous system of the heart. These effects depend upon the intensity and duration of application.

Reaction Phase:

Slowing down of the heart beat with the active dilatation of the small vessels. Arterial tension remains elevated.

A. Short cold application over the chest area:

> Stimulate the activity of the heart.

> Increase the arterial tension.

i.e. cold applied for a shorter duration brings about following changes:

> Produce brief contraction of the visceral vessels followed by dilatation for 3 – 10 min. This ends up with the contraction of the vessels. Blood pressure remains constantly raised throughout this vascular phenomenon.

Therefore short cold applications over the heart are tonic in its effects as it increases the force of contraction and blood pressure.

Short general cold application is also a potent tonic for the heart.

B. Prolonged (3 -10 min) general cold or cool applications:

> Slows down the heart beat with the elevation of the blood pressure.

C. Effects of local cold application:

They are of two types: 1. Reflex effect

2. Direct effect

1. **Plethysmographic experiments by Franck**

   Ice held in one hand

   Observations:

   - Contraction of the vessels in other hand (in 2 to 3 seconds)
   - Changes return to normal within a minute.

2. **Compensatory Effect of cold: Findings of Winternitz**

   Observations:

   - Immersion of the elbow in water at 50° F for ½ an hour
   - Increased axillary temperature (increase in the internal temperature)
   - Simultaneous reduction in external temperature.

3. **Cold over the trunk of an artery**

   Observations:

   - Ice application over elbow/ knee
   - Contraction in its distal branches.

     (Reduced blood flow in the arm/ leg)

4. **Very cold compress**

   Observations:

   - Ice compress over the throat

   - Reduces cerebral blood flow

5. **Observations of Winternitz**

   Observations:

   - Cold applications to limited skin surface

   - Increased pulse (for 3 minutes)

   - Sow reduction of Pulse

EFFECTS OF COLD ON RESPIRATION:

1. **Effect on breathing movements**

2. **Effect on exchange of gases**

1. Effect on breathing movements:

a. Application of percutient measures:

General cold douche produces quick & gasping breathing.

Local cold douche

Action phase: with application to the chest or upper part of the body subject experiences constriction in the chest. There is short, gasping respiration observed.

Reaction Phase: Breathing becomes slower and deeper with enhanced absorption of oxygen. Uneasy sensation disappears in the chest.

Note:

The sudden application of cold to the chest causes constriction of the pulmonary vessels due to which the volume of blood available for gaseous exchange will be reduced. But the demand for the exchange of gases remains high. This leads to the gasping of respiration.

b. Application of non percutient measures: Cold immersion bath

Action Phase: Initial slowing of the respiration

Reaction Phase: Deeper and slower breathing. Increase in the tidal air.

2. Effect on exchange of gases: Cold applications increase

- ✓ Oxygen absorption
- ✓ Carbon dioxide elimination

Note:

- ❖ Experiments of Crawford showed that tissue oxidation increases with the cold applications as evidenced by the difference in the colour of the arterial and venous blood.

- ❖ Observations of Leibig confirmed increase of tissue activity with the exposure to cold air, cold water and exercise.

❖ When the body is exposed to a temperature of 40°F (4°C) or lesser produces shivering due to increased heat production and CO_2 elimination also increased.

EFFECTS OF COLD UPON MUSCLES:

1. **Effect on voluntary muscles**
2. **Effect on involuntary muscles**

1. Effect on voluntary muscles

Mode of application	Voluntary muscles
Prolonged cold at low temperature	Decrease muscle energy & irritability
Short local cold application	Increase the energy & excitability
Short general cold application	Increase the energy & excitability

Table 8: Summary of effects of cold on voluntary muscles

Note: increased muscle tone causes shivering in cold exposure. Short (1to 2sec) cold bath with high pressure (25 to 35 lbs) produces Restorative effect (Fatigue)

2. Effect on involuntary muscles:

Mode of application	Involuntary muscles
General or local cold application	a. Excites smooth muscle fibres of the skin(goose flesh appearance) b. Contracts smooth muscles of the small blood vessels
Application over reflex areas (feet, lower abdomen)	Excites the involuntary muscles of the related internal viscera. (bowel, bladder)
• **Cold spray to feet** • **Stepping in to cold bath**	Shivering & goose flesh appearance throughout the body.
• **Cold spray to one half of the body**	Causes goose flesh appearance on the other half of the body.

Table 9: Effect of cold on involuntary muscles

EFFECTS OF COLD ON NERVOUS SYSTEM:

Nerve impulse transmission:

✓ Findings of Helmholtz showed reduced nerve impulse transmission with the cold application to a nerve. With removal of application nerve regains its normal function.

✓ When the application is prolonged and strong even after its removal nerve sensibility remains high. A sensation of pain is felt in the area of nerve distribution.

Cerebral activity:

1. Short cold application to the head:

Action phase: brief period of reduced cerebral activity which remains unnoticed because of the intense reaction.

Reaction phase: increased cerebral activity.

2. Prolonged very cold application to the head: Diminishes the cerebral activity. Leads to drowsiness.

Reflex effects of cold applications

Hydrotherapy practitioners like Edward, Winternitz and Franck studied the reflex effects of cold.

Cold application to a cutaneous area produces both local and distant effects. These effects observed in the distant parts or organs are called as reflex effects.

There are two types of reflex areas, they are:

1. Muscular reflex areas

2. Special Skin reflex areas (to internal organs)

1. Muscular reflex areas: Application of cold to certain areas produces contraction in the certain muscle groups.

S. NO	Muscular reflex areas
1.	The interscapular area (space between the shoulder blades)
2.	The epigastric area (the sides of the chest at the level of the 4th rib)
3.	The abdominal area (the borders of the recti muscles)
4.	The cremasteric area (the inner and upper surface of the thighs)
5.	The plantar area (the sole of the foot)

Table 10: Muscular reflex areas

By the stimulation of these specific areas many muscle groups are activated.eg: A jet of cold or very hot water (Extremes of temperature have the similar physiological effects) application to the abdomen causes sudden and intense contraction of the abdominal muscles which in turn stimulates intestinal peristalsis.

Short, intense cold application with strong pressure on these areas enhance the nutrition of the related muscles.

Indications of reflex applications (muscular reflex areas):

- General muscle weakness
- Paresis, paralysis
- Progressive muscular atrophy
- Conditions which include wasting of muscles

2. Special Skin reflex areas: The vessels of the internal organs are influenced to contract or dilate by the cold applications made on the special skin areas.

a. Short and intense applications (duration: 1 to 4 sec, temp: 40° to 60°F, pressure: 25 to 35lbs) produce dilatation in the visceral vessels.

b. Long and moderate applications produce contraction in the corresponding visceral vessels.

c. Application of cold to a reflex area produces a sensation of constriction in the related internal organ.

For eg: Cold douche to the feet causes sense of constriction in the lower abdomen.

Cold to the chest causes constricting sensation in the thorax.

List of internal organs and corresponding skin reflex areas

S. NO.	Skin reflex area	Corresponding Internal organ
1.	**head, neck, face, hands and feet**	Brain
2.	**neck, face, upper dorsal spine, hands and feet**	Nasal mucous membrane
3.	**lower dorsal spine, epigastrium**	Stomach

4.	lumbar region, lower portion of the sternum, feet	Kidney
5.	Feet and abdomen	Bowels
6.	feet and lower abdomen	Bladder
7.	lower right chest	Liver
8.	lower left chest	Spleen
9.	chest and the thighs, upper dorsal region	Lungs
10.	lumbar region, breast, abdomen, inner surface of the thighs, the feet, cervix uteri through the vagina.	Uterus

Table 11: List of skin reflex areas & related internal organs

Following are the various applications recommended in the treatment of different conditions:

S. No.	Condition	Application	Mechanism
1.	**Cerebral hyperaemia**	Prolonged cold arm bath	Contraction of the vessels of the brain and nasal mucous membrane.
		Prolonged cold head pour	Contraction of the vessels of the brain

2.	**Uterine hemorrhage**	prolonged cool foot bath cold lumbar douche at moderate pressure (15to 45 secs.)	Contraction of the uterine vessels
		Prolonged cold to the breast and inner thighs	Contraction of the vessels and muscles of the uterus.
		Short very cold to the hands	Contraction of the uterine muscles.
3.	**Amenorrhoea**	Short very cold douche to the feet with strong pressure (25-35lbs) Very cold very short douche (2 to 4 secs.) with strong pressure (25 to 35 lbs) to the lumbar area	Dilatation of uterine vessels
		Prolonged Ice compress or ice bag to the lumbar region	Dilatation of the vessels of the uterus and lower extremities
4.	**Epistaxis**	Prolonged cold to the upper dorsal region	Xontraction of the vessels of nasal mucous membrane
5.	**Pulmonary congestion and hemorrhage**	Prolonged cold to the upper dorsal and lower cervical region	Contraction of pulmonary vessels.

6.	**Tachycardia**	Prolonged cold to the occiput and the neck	Sedates the heart
7.	**To increase the urine output**	Short cold douche to the lower portion of sternum	Stimulates kidneys
8.	**To stimulate the activity of abdominal organs**	Short cold douche with strong pressure to the skin over liver, spleen, stomach, bowels etc	Dilatation of the corresponding blood vessels.
9.	**Relieve congestion and lessen the activity of an organ**	Prolonged cold to the skin overlying the internal organs without pressure	Contraction of the corresponding blood vessels
10.	**To enhance concentration and alertness**	Short cold to the face and neck	Dilatation of the cerebral vessels

Table 12: Cold Application over reflex areas in therapy

EFFECTS OF COLD UPON THE BLOOD CELLS

S. NO.	Scientist	Application	Findings
1.	**Winternitz (1893)**	General cold	Increase the number of RBC, WBC and Hb concentration in the general circulation.

2.	**Kellog**	Local cold	Increase the blood cells and Hb levels at the site of application without increase in other areas.
3.	**Henocque**	Cold & hot	Increase in the reduced oxyhemoglobin
4.	**Crawford (England, 1781)**	Cold baths	Increase of colour contrast between the arterial and venous blood. (increase the oxidation and tissue activity)
5.	**D'Arsonval and others**	General Cold	Increase gaseous exchange in the lungs
6.	**Strasser**	General Cold	Increase in the alkalinity of blood

Table 13: Observations of Effects of Cold on blood cells

EFFECTS OF COLD ON ABSORPTION, SECRETION & NUTRITION

S. No	Application	Effect
1.	**General cold**	Increased absorption from the gut

2.	**Short general cold & prolonged cold.**	Stimulate the glandular activity in stomach, liver, kidney & other secretary organs.
3.	**Short general cold to skin**	Enhances vital functions, blood & lymph flow, absorption & disintegration. Increases vital resistance

Table 14: Effects of cold on absorption & secretion

Experiment by Fleury

Experiments conducted by Fleury and others concluded that cold douche to the surface stimulated absorption from the alimentary canal. As a result nutrition of the part was enhanced.

Belladonna was introduced in to the rectum of the subject and the time taken for pupilary dilatation and physiological changes to appear was noted. The same was done along with the general Cold douche. Application of cold douche greatly enhanced absorption from the alimentary canal as evidenced by the lesser time taken for pupilary dilatation.

Experiment by Strasser

Strasser observed the increased absorption of phosphates from food on application of cold to the surface and increased elimination in the form of earthy phosphates. This fact was beneficial in the treatment of rickets as increased absorption of phosphates contributes to the development of healthy bones.

Short very cold douche with the high pressure (25 to 35 lbs) to the stomach and liver stimulated secretory function in these organs. This was due to the vasodilatation effect produced with the application. Thus secretary cells activity was stimulated.

Experiment by J. H. Kellogg

A cold percussion douche (55°F) to the epigastrium and to the spine opposite for two minutes increased the hydrochloric acid in the gastric secretion. Thus the application is indicated in hypopepsia.

Note:

General cod douche increases the HCL secretion.

Alternate circle douche enhances the secretion of peptic juice.

EFFECT OF COLD ON EXCRETION AND TISSUE CHANGE

S. No	Application	Effect
1.	**Short general cold to skin**	Stimulate perspiration by dilatation of surface vessels. Increase the CO_2 excretion and O_2 absorption (Increase heat production)

2.	**Prolonged cold**	Reduce perspiration & CO2 excretion (Reduce heat production).
4.	**Cold douche to lower 1/3rd of sternum**	Stimulates renal function.
5.	**Cold immersion**	Increase urine formation with increase in total solids.

Table 15: Effect of cold on excretion and tissue change

Note:

The toxic content in the urine is increased by six fold when fever cases are treated with cold bath. Therefore cold baths enhance the renal function.

Experiment by Strasser

Studies of Strasser revealed that cold baths excite the process of tissue change within the body. This was proved by increased the amount of urea, uric acid, ammonia, earthy phosphates, xanthine bases and the total nitrogen produced on short cold (tonic) applications.

Cold applications reduced the amount of imperfectly oxidized extractives to 1.5% which amounted for 8.7% prior to the application. This signifies the stimulation of oxidation process under the influence of cold.

EFFECT OF COLD ON TEMPERATURE

S. No	Application	Effect
1.	**General cold**	Decrease Skin & general temperature
2.	**Cold spray to the soles of the feet**	Reduces general temperature
3.	**Cold to the head**	Reduces general temperature (depressing action on thermogenic centres)
4.	**Short Cold**	Stimulate heat production
5.	**Prolonged cold**	First increase then reduce the heat production

Table 16: Effect of cold on temperature

Note: According to Gautrelet cold application to the surface enhances the thermoelectrical phenomenon. (Conversion of thermal energy into electrical energy). Enhancing thermoelectrical currents within the body modifies storage & discharge of nervous energy. This special area needs further investigations.

Cold bath influences the reduction of body temperature. This effect is more pronounced when the application is more cold and of longer duration. **These changes in temperature will be more marked in febrile states than the normal circumstances.** Body surface continues to remain cold even after the reaction which is seen by reddening of the skin. This indicates that the cooling of the blood is continued.

The reduction of body temperature is increased with the application of friction to the body during the bath. Friction maintains the surface circulation by drawing more blood towards the skin which is cooled continuously.

- Winternitz showed that friction in the cold bath increases the rate of heat elimination by 30% and

- Pospichil noted an increase of more than 44%.

Note:

1. Shivering produced in cold applications is due to

    - Reduced internal temperature
    - Beginning of increase in heat production

2. Circulatory reaction in cold: produced by reflex effect on the vasomotor centres & direct effect on visceral sympathetic ganglia in the blood vessels.

Thermic reaction of cold: Produced by reduction in skin & blood temperature.

Evidences:

- ❖ Currie concluded that cold application to the surface reduce both surface and internal body temperature.

❖ Fleury observed reduction of 7°F after the cold immersion bath at 50°F for 25 minutes. He was the first to observe that body temperature doesn't begin to fall for sometime after the removal from the bath.

❖ Observations of Jurgensen showed 6.5°F decrease in the temperature after the cold bath.

Effect of Local cold application on the body temperature:

- Water temperatures below the body temperature decreases the temperature of the area of application.

- Immersion of a hand or foot in cold water (circumscribed applications) decrease the temperature at the area of application. They do not influence the general temperature.

- Winternitz observed snow application to forearm reduces the hand temperature initially (2°F) & then increases (1.3°F).

- Holding of ice in the mouth reduces the temperature of the cheek on the same side.

- Drinking large amount of ice water reduces the temperature of skin over the epigastrium.

Local applications which reduce the general temperature:

✓ Cold compress to the trunk (when larger area is involved),

- ✓ Ice cap to the head (depressing the activity of thermogenic centres.)
- ✓ Ice bag application over the heart (slows the circulation and cools the blood.)
- ✓ Drinking large quantities of cold water reduction of general temperature & Large cold water enema more prominent in fever

Influence of prolonged cold applications on reaction:

Cold application for prolonged duration suppresses the reaction because of the continuous influence of cold stimulus.

Mechanism of cooling effect in prolonged cold applications

- Prolonged application of cold reduces the sensibility of nerves
- Exhausts the nerve centres and
- Exhausts the powers of calorification (power of heat production).

  Thus body fails to overcome the depressing effect of cold. So antithermic (cooling) effects will be produced.

When the application of cold is long continued then the thermal and vital activities of the body are suppressed as indicated by the delay (two to three hours) in attaining the normal body temperature.

An English investigator **Edward** has shown in his experiments that it requires longer time to restore the body temperature after repetitive cooling of an animal. Hence this property of cold water had found a great value in treating typhoid fevers.

PHYSIOLOGICAL EFFECTS OF HEAT

Sources of heat in therapeutic applications: hot water, hot air, steam, radiation from incandescent light.

Modes of heat application: Full bath, fomentation, Russian bath, vapor bath, vapor douche, Turkish bath, hot air bath and electric light bath.

Factors influencing the effects of heat on the body are:

1. Condition of the patient

2. Mode, Temperature & Duration of application.

Range of temperature used in Therapy:

Temperature	°F	°C
Hot	98 – 104	37 -40
Very hot	›104	40 & above
Russian bath	112 - 120	44 - 49
Turkish bath	140 – 180	60 - 82

Table 17: Therapeutic range of temperature

General physiological effects of heat application:

- Expansion of the white fibrous tissue is seen. Ligaments are relaxed with the heat application as they are made up of white fibrous tissue.

- Contraction of the yellow elastic tissue is observed.

- Heat stimulates cellular activities, therapeutic use of poultice or fomentation for long duration stimulates skin pigmentation.

Effects of heat on specific systems and organs:

Effect of heat on the skin, blood cells and its circulation, respiration, muscles, nervous system, tissue nutrition and excretion, digestion, thermoregulation etc will have varied effects.

EFFECTS OF HEAT ON THE SKIN

The effects of heat application on the skin differ according to the intensity and the modality of application. Generally the effects are as follows: -

1. **Dilatation of the capillaries**
2. **Stimulation of the cutaneous secretion and excretion**
3. **Enhanced heat loss by the skin**
4. **Diminished tactile sensibility**
5. **Preparation of the skin for the cold application**

1. Dilatation of the capillaries:

Currie's observation on heat application at different temperatures:

Water temperature	Temp. Range	Effect on surface vesssels
Moderate Heat	99 ° to 101°F	Vasodilatation
Very Hot	104°F & More	Vasoconstriction
High Heat	110° to 130°F	Short VC followed by VD Brief period of pallor then dusky redness of skin.

Table 18: Observation of Currie on different range of heat application

* VC: VasoConstriciton, VD: VasoDilatation

Note: In gradual applications of heat starting from moderate heat (100° to 104°F) & then reaching up to 130°F or higher initial excitation of the vasoconstrictors is not seen instead the surface remains reddened.

If the hot application is continued from 15 to 30 minutes vasoconstriction can occur at the end of the application in some cases.

1. The effect of heat on the circulation of the mucous membrane remains same as that of the skin. Slightly higher temperature applied to the mucous membrane produces the same effects.

2. The vasoconstricting effect of higher temperature (120° to 160°F) can be utilized to stop bleeding and in capillary oozing of surgical wounds.

3. To stop bleeding in menorrhagia Kellogg used a hollow uterine sound through which a stream of hot water(170°F) was passed.

4. Along with the dilatation of the arteries hot application to the skin produces dilatation of the small veins and lymphatic vessels.

2. Stimulation of the cutaneous secretion and excretion:

Cutaneous secretion: General or local application of heat to the skin increases the activity of perspiratory and sebaceous glands. Degree of perspiration may vary from producing slight moist skin to profuse sweating according to the length and intensity of application.

Normally one to one and half ounce of moisture is thrown out of the skin per hour. This rate increases up to 50 to 60 times the normal rate in very hot applications (110° to 115°F).i.e more than an ounce a minute. Electric light bath and the Sun bath produces more pronounced effects.

Cutaneous respiration: Normally skin performs one percent of respiratory work out of the whole work done by the respiratory system. This is doubled with hot application. Hot application increases the oxygen absorption and carbon dioxide elimination from the skin while the same is reduced from the lungs.

Increased cutaneous respiration of the skin is evident by the dilatation of skin vessels and moistening of the horny layer facilitating exchange of gases.

3. Enhanced heat loss by the skin: Hot application increases the heat loss through the skin in the following ways:

1. Dilating the surface vessels, increases the volume of blood exposed to cooling effect of environmental air.

2. Stimulation of the heart and vasodilators increases the rate of blood flow through the skin vessels.

3. Heating of the skin, stimulation of sweat glands and increased osmosis all account for increased evaporation from the skin surface.

4. Increased conductivity of the skin increases the loss of heat by radiation.

4. Diminished tactile sensibility: Very hot application (113°F & more) decreases the touch sensibility.

Eg: A 23 year old subject felt 2 points on the back of the hand at a distance of 20mm on asthesiometer. After immersion of hand in water of 117°F for four & half minutes he could distinguish 2 points at 30mm distance.

Water application between 98°F to 95°F produced no change in the tactile sensibility.

Note: Tactile sensibility of the skin is greatest at 95° to 98° F i.e at normal surface temperature.

5. Preparation of the skin for the cold application: Hot application prior to the cold application has great therapeutic significance. Prior hot applications increase the skin temperature and stimulate vascular & nervous activity. So they prepare the skin for further cold applications and to produce more powerful reaction.

Indications of pre heating the skin before cold applications:

cold skin, fatigue, rheumatism with joint pain, neuralgia, anemia & in feeble patients.

EFFECTS OF HEAT UPON THE CIRCULATION

Heat application increases both cardiac and vascular activity of the skin.

The heart: General application of heat initially increases the arterial pressure and transient slowing of pulse rate. As the perspiration started the arterial pressure reduced and pulse rate increased.

Final effect: General heat application reduces arterial tension and increases the pulse rate.

The skin: Application of heat to the skin causes following changes:

Stimulation of the vasoconstrictors of the skin causes transient stimulation of the heart. This leads to the following changes:

> Stimulation of the vasoconstrictors: temporary contraction of internal blood vessels with the contraction of the small blood vessels on the surface.

> This is immediately followed by pronounced dilatation of the vessels.

> When the surface vessels are relaxed considerably this leads to contraction again.

> Transient stimulation of the heart with the stimulation of skin vasoconstrictors causes congestion in the internal organs specially the brain. This produces throbbing sensation and fullness in the head, noticeable pulsations in the throat, temple and flushing of the cheeks.

> Hot applications are contra indicated to persons with plethora, apoplexy, and arteriosclerosis.

EFFECTS OF HEAT ON RESPIRATION

General applications of heat:

> Increase the rate of respiration

> Facilitate easy movements of respiration

> Depth of respiration is reduced i.e the amount of tidal air is reduced.

Mechanism of general applications of heat:

Increase in blood temperature

↓

Stimulation of heat controlling centers

↓

Beginning of heat dissipation

- **Increased lung activity**
- **Increased skin perspiration**
- **Increased skin respiration**

After the bath:

> Transient reduction in rate and depth of respiration is observed.

Note: Full Immersion bath at high temperatures between 110° to 112°F causes a sense of constriction in the chest an effect similar to that of cold. Walls of the abdomen are contracted. These effects are more pronounced with applications of douche with high pressure.

EFFECTS OF HEAT ON MUSCLES

1. Very short hot applications Restorative effect

> Very Short hot applications relieve the exhaustion induced by prolonged exercise. A person in the

state of exhaustion will not respond to cold hence there is a necessity for hot applications.

> More pronounced effects will be observed if the hot application is succeeded by cold application in the form of

- Broken cold horizontal jet to the spine for 3 to 4 seconds
- Rubbing wet sheet
- Cold friction bath

To obtain better restorative effect apply hot bath for more than 5 minutes follow it with a cold shower or spray douche for 5 to 20 seconds and end with a very cold broken douche to the spine for 2 seconds.

Mechanism: The restorative effects of hot are due to

- Enhanced elimination of the fatigue poisons and
- Reflex stimulation of nerve centers.

2. High temperatures reduce irritability of voluntary muscles:

Hot application at 120°F and above quickly lessen the irritability of muscles.

Very prolonged hot applications with the temperatures slightly above the normal body temperature produces muscle weakness in human beings.

Indications of very hot applications to reduce the muscle irritability:

- Deformities resulting from muscular contraction, vaginismus, contraction of anal muscle.

Prolonged neutral full bath (92°to 95°F) is indicated in conditions of

- Excess muscular irritations like cramps, fidgets and muscular twitching.

3. High temperatures increase irritability of involuntary muscles

Very hot applications to the skin causes contraction of the blood vessels which are made up of smooth muscles and contraction of the muscles connected with the hair bulbs. This produces pallor and goose flesh appearance of the skin.

Indications:

- Application of hot water to the uterus through vaginal injection is given in conditions of hemorrhage and sub involution.

- Application of hot rectal irrigation for chronic congestion and enlarged prostate.

- A large hot enema or coloclyster to relieve constipation when other means are ineffective.

EFFECTS OF HEAT ON THE TEMPERATURE

General application:

Experiments of Kellogg have concluded that Immersion bath at the body temperature for one hour increases the temperature by 1.8°F.

Immersion bath at 104° F for 15 minutes increases the body temperature by 3-4° F.

Short hot applications: They reduce the heat production and increase the elimination of heat. Increased heat elimination is evident by increased sweating, vasodilatation of the surface vesssels and stimulation of the heart activity.

Prolonged hot application: increase the body temperature by reducing the heat loss and stimulating the heat production.

Prolonged hot bath few degrees higher than the normal body temperature causes increased heat production and heat accumulation causing threatening levels of body temperature.

EFFECTS OF HEAT ON THE NERVOUS SYSTEM

Excitation & Exhaustion: Baths at 100°F & above produce excitation of the nervous system. This is evident by nervousness, headache etc. Later on it exhausts the system.

Reduced nervous irritability: Baths at neutral temperature (92°– 95°F, for 30 min to one & half an hour) reduce nervous irritability. Therefore they produce sedative effect.

Stimulation of protoplasmic activity: Hot applications stimulate the protoplasmic activity. This produces accumulation of tissue waste which resembles building up of fatigue poisons after violent exercises and this is the cause of exhaustion produced in hot baths.

Reflex effects of hot application: Application of hot on special regions on the skin produce changes in the connected internal organs.

- Warm and hot application causes vasodilatation.
- Very hot (115° to 130°F) causes vasoconstriction.

Remarkable work was made on the study of exact skin surfaces which have to be operated to produce the desired effect. Winternitz, Brown –Sequard, Tholozan, Rosbach & others are the pioneers in this work. **Refer Table 11 for reflex areas &related internal organs.**

Clinical applications of Reflex effect:

1. Hot foot bath at 105° to 110°F relieves cerebral congestion.
2. Hot full bath at 102°F reduces cerebral hyperemia.

3. Very hot water application to the face stops nose bleeding.

4. Hot sponging of the head and neck relieves insomnia due to cerebral congestion.

5. Very hot sponging over the back of the neck relieves congestive headache.

6. Very hot fomentation over the area of liver & spleen relieves the congestion of these organs as seen in malaria.

7. Short very hot foot bath at 105° to 115°F stops uterine bleeding.

EFFECTS OF HEAT ON BLOOD

1. Experiment by Winternitz & others noted following observations with the hot water applications:

➤ Reduction in the blood count due to the retention of blood cells in the visceral organs.

➤ Reduction in the Hb percentage in relation to reduced red blood cells.

➤ Hot applied to a circumscribed area increases the number of white blood cells and diminishes red blood cells in the area.

2. Experiments by Henoque showed reduction in oxyhemoglobin. **These physiological changes might induce mottled skin appearance following hot applications.**

3. Experiments of Strasser noted following changes:

> General hot applications reduce the alkalinity of blood as a result of increase in the acid phosphate level double than the normal.

EFFECTS OF HEAT ON NUTRITION

> Heat application to the body excites the entire structures in the body. So there is stimulation of the cellular activity without increasing the oxygen absorption.

> Oxidation is reduced as evidenced by the reduction in oxygen absorption and CO_2 exhalation.

> Greater reduction in the oxidation might result in increased blood sugar levels and its passage in urine.

> **Precaution: Great care has to be taken on delivering hot applications to diabetics and patients with reduced oxidation.**

> Nitrogen elimination is increased in the form of uric acid.

> Regular heat application to the skin stimulates pigment cells. Sunlight & electric light bath also produces same effect.

THE EFFECTS OF HEAT ON DIGESTIVE ORGANS

1. Stomach:

Measures to increase HCl secretion: Fomentation over the area of stomach for an hour or two after food.

Measures to decrease HCl secretion (in hyperpepsia):

1. Hot douche to the stomach area & opposite spinal area.

2. General hot bath.

2. Liver:

Measures to stimulate the activity of liver & flow of bile: Hot compress or fomentation over the area of liver.

3. Intestine, pancreas & spleen:

Fomentation over the abdomen stimulate the function of the intestines, pancreas & spleen.

THE EFFECTS OF HEAT ON BODY TEMPERATURE AND HEAT PRODUCTION

1. General heat applications: Immediate increase of body temperature.

Immersion bath at body temperature for one hour: increases body temperature by 1.8°F

Immersion bath at 104°F: 3° to 4° F increase of temperature within 15 minutes.

Modern Calorimetric findings reveal that:

Short heat application to the body reduce heat production & increase heat elimination as evidenced by increased sweating, increased activity of heart and relaxation of the surface blood vessels. This is atonic reaction that follows heat application.

Prolonged heat application: increases body temperature by reducing heat elimination and increasing heat production.

Note:

> **Conditions that cause increase of body temperature increases heat production.**

> **Conditions that increase heat elimination tends to increase heat production.**

ORGANIC CHANGES PRODUCED BY COLD AND HEAT APPLICATION

> Short cold applications increase the body temperature and metabolism.

> Prolonged cold applications reduce the body temperature and metabolism.

> Short hot applications reduce the temperature and metabolism.

> Prolonged hot applications increase the temperature and metabolism; they also increase the oxidation of albumin.

> At neutral applications body temperature and metabolism remains normal.

SUMMARY OF COLD & HEAT APPLICATIONS

S. NO	APPLICATION	COLD	HEAT
1.	General: a. Primary	Depressant	Stimulant
	b. Short	Excitant by tonic reaction Reflex dilatation of visceral vessels	Depressant by atonic reaction Reflex fluxion & derivative effect
	c. Prolonged	Depressant	Mixed(stimulant & depressant
2.	Skin a. Action	Reduced activity Local anemia, collateral hyperemia	Increased activity Local hyperemia, collateral anemia
	b. Reaction	Increased activity Local hyperemia, collateral anemia	Reduced activity Local anemia, collateral hyperemia
	c. Sensibility	Lessened	Lessened
3.	Heart	First quickens then slows, Force increased	First slows, then quickens Force reduced
4.	Blood Vessels a. Action	Contraction	Contraction then Dilatation
	b. Reaction	Dilatation	Contraction
	c. Tone & activity	Increased	Decreased, activity reduced
5.	Nerves	Benumbs & paralyzes Excites by tonic reaction	Excitation Depresses by atonic reaction

6.	Muscles a. Short	Increased excitability & capacity	Lessens fatigue
	b. Prolonged	Reduced excitability & capacity	Reduced excitability & capacity
7.	Lungs	Slow & deep breathing Increased respired air Increased Co2 Increased respiratory quotient	Quick & easy breathing Reduced respired air Decreased CO2 Reduced respiratory quotient
8.	Stomach	Increased HCl & motor activity	Decreased HCl & motor activity
9.	Kidney	Congestion & excitation	Anemic & reduces activity
10.	Heat production a. short	Increased	Reduced
	b. prolonged	Reduced	Increased
11.	Blood count	Increased, especially WBC	Decreased RBC, Increased WBC
12.	Metabolism	Increased CO2 & urea Improved oxidation	Decreased CO2, increased urea & proteid waste.

Table 19: Summary of cold & heat application

THERAPEUTIC EFFECTS OF HYDROTHERAPY APPLICATIONS

Hydrotherapeutic applications are capable of producing wide range of effects. Observations of hydrotherapy practitioners have revealed that an identical application may be exciting or sedative under different set of circumstances. This feature is applicable not only to water but to different therapeutic agents. This is because of the fact that no two individuals are alike and the internal state varies at every moment. In spite of these fluctuations under the standard set of conditions practitioners could derive definite outcomes. This provides the basis for the classification of the hydrotherapeutic effects.

06

Classification of Hydriatic Effects

In general therapeutic effects of water are grouped into two major categories. They are:

1. EXCITANT

2. SEDATIVE

Each one is further classified into different subdivisions.

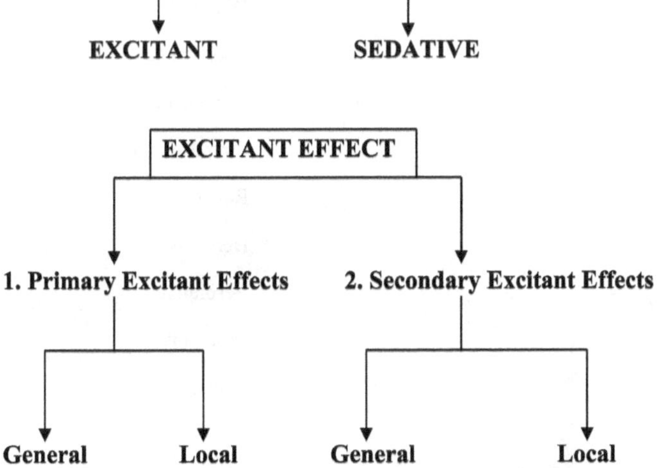

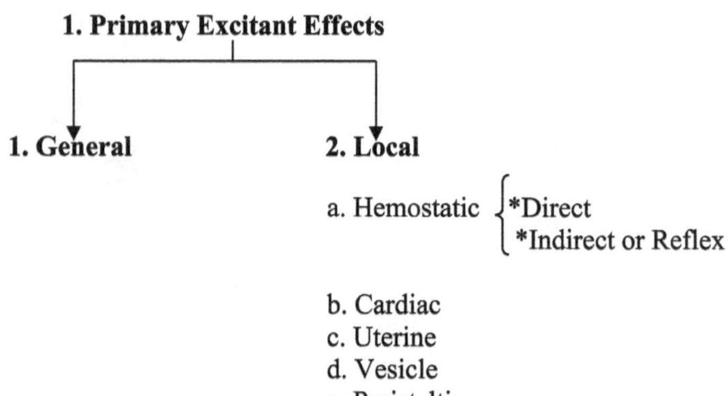
1. Primary Excitant Effects
1. General
2. Local
a. Hemostatic
*Direct
*Indirect or Reflex
b. Cardiac
c. Uterine
d. Vesicle
e. Peristaltic

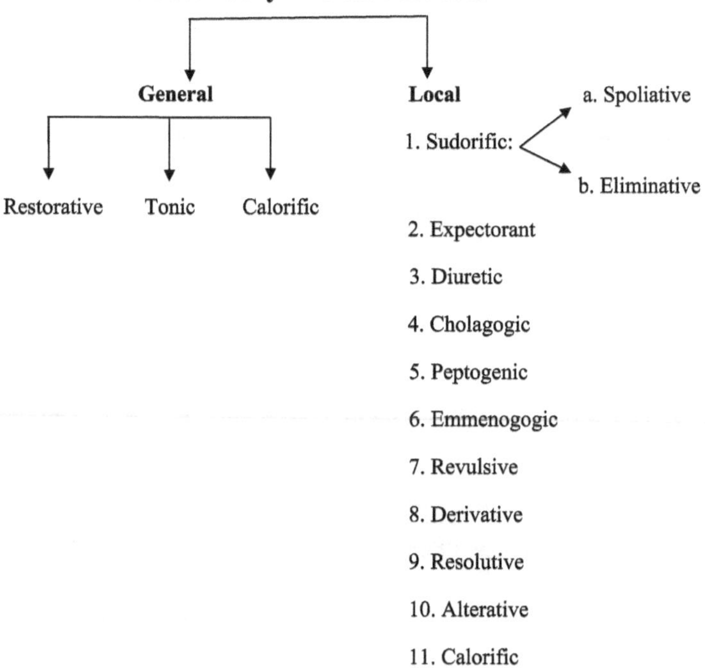
2. Secondary Excitant Effects
General
Local
Restorative
Tonic
Calorific
1. Sudorific:
a. Spoliative
b. Eliminative
2. Expectorant
3. Diuretic
4. Cholagogic
5. Peptogenic
6. Emmenogogic
7. Revulsive
8. Derivative
9. Resolutive
10. Alterative
11. Calorific

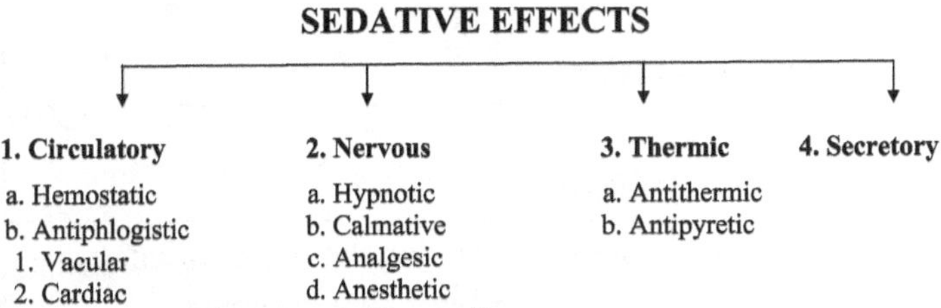

GENERAL PRINCIPLES OF HOT, COLD & NEUTRAL WATER APPLICATIONS:

S. NO	WATER TEMPERATURE	PRIMARY EFFECT	SECONDARY EFFECT
1.	Hot	Excitant	Depressant, Sedative, Tonic
2.	Cold	Sedative	Invigorating, Restorative, Tonic
3.	Neutral	No Change	Calmative, Restorative

Table 20: General Principles of Hot, Cold & Neutral Water Applications

EFFECT OF HOT APPLICATION:

Effect of hot water application depends upon multiple factors, they are:

1. **Condition of the patient**

2. **Intensity & Length of the application**

3. **Form of application**

S. NO	FORM OF HOT APPLICATTION	EFFECT
1.	Very short, very high temperature	Excitant
2.	Slightly prolonged, less intense	During the application: Moderate excitation, After the application: Depressant & atonic effect.
3.	Prolonged & at high temperature	Both Excitant & Depressant

Table 21: Summary of effect of hot application

Note: In prolonged heat application excitation is due to increased body temperature and depression due to exhaustion of nervous system respectively.

EFFECT OF COLD APPLICATION:

Effect of cold water application depends upon multiple factors, they are:

1. **Method of application**

2. **Temperature of application**

3. **Susceptibility & condition of the patient**

S. NO	FORM OF COLD APPLICATION	EFFECT
1.	Short, intense cold	Excitant, if repeated daily tonic

2.	More prolonged, moderately low temperature	Less excitant, Less tonic
3.	Prolonged Cold application	Initially excitant then sedative

Table 22: Effect of Cold Application

Note: Effect of bath (hot or cold) can be enhanced by following measures:

1. **Addition of mechanical effect like percussion. E.g.: through douche, friction with the hand, towel or sheet.**

2. **Measures which enhance or delay the reaction: by applications given before, during or after the bath. E.g.: Exercise, artificial heat.**

EFFECT OF NEUTRAL APPLICATION:

Effect of neutral application differs than that of the hot or cold application. Following are the characteristics changes produced:

1. **No Reaction:** Neutral bath (92° to 95°F) does not produce any reaction. Either thermic or circulatory.

2. **Calmative Effect:** Reduces the sensibility of cutaneous nerves & thus suppresses reflex activity. This results in calmative effect of neutral application.

3. **Restorative Effect:** Neutral application checks the loss of energy and enhances renal and cutaneous activity.

Note: Applications with the intermediate temperature produce mixed effect. Prominent effect depends upon the temperature of water to which it is closer to (cold, hot or neutral)

EXCITANT EFFECTS: These effects are action phase of thermic applications which are reflex in nature. They are of two types:

1. **Primary Excitant effects**
    1. **General Primary Excitant effects**
    2. **Local Primary Excitant effects**
2. **Secondary Excitant effects**

1. PRIMARY EXCITANT EFFECTS:

Introduction:

Instant effect produced by the application of cold or hot on the skin or mucous membrane are called as primary excitant effects.

Duration of application:

- Short, from 2or 3 sec. to 1or 2 min.
- Shorter the application more pronounced will be the excitant effect.

Temperature of application:

- Hot or cold applications produce the excitant effects.

- Very cold or very hot applications are more excitant than cold, cool or hot or warm applications.

- strong excitant effect will be produced with the greater temperature difference between the skin & that of application with regard to both cold & hot applications.

1. General Primary Excitant effects:

- General applications produce the general excitant effects.

- Local applications like hot enema, hot sitz bath, hot to the head and spine, very hot applications to the heart also produce excitant effects.

- Sun bath & electric light bath produce powerful excitant effects.

General Measures to produce the excitant effects are as follows:

S. NO	MEASURES	TEMPERATURE	DURATION
1.	Very hot douche or shower, Spray or jet	110° -130°F	15 seconds to 4 minutes

2.	Very hot affusion	110° -115°F	30 sec. to 5 min.
3.	Hot blanket pack	105° – 112°F	5 to 10 min.
4.	Hot water drinking, general alternate hot & cold sponging, full bath	105°- 110°F	5 to 10 min.

Table 23: General measures for excitant effects

Note:

- Alternate applications should be applied for equal duration (15 seconds each)

- Strongest excitant effect is produced with alternate douche.

- Alternate hot &cold sponging, compress, affusions also produce powerful excitant effects.

Alternate applications are the best exciting measures for the following reasons: Short heat application followed by cold application of equal length arouses the nerve centers initially under the influence of short hot application. A short cold application succeeded by the hot restores the skin temperature to normal & prepares the skin for next exciting application (hot).

Since both the applications are shorter reaction will be suppressed by succeeding application.

Indications of general excitant measures:

1. Extreme exhaustion

2. Collapse

3. Surgical shock

4. Collapse under anesthesia

5. Drowning

6. Suffocation

7. Syncope from hemorrhage

8. Fright

Note: Heat application is the measure of choice over cold application in case of collapse or pain. Application should be short and followed by a very cold application to overcome the depressing effect of heat.

Contra indications:

General very hot applications are avoided in following conditions:

1. Arteriosclerosis

2. Weak heart

3. Advanced age

4. Children (less than 7 years)

5. History of sun stroke or heat stroke

Precautions:

- In Hot applications made over the large skin areas ice cap or cold compress should be applied to the head area to prevent cerebral excitation

- Care must be taken to avoid over excitation of the heart.

2. Local Primary Excitant effects:

a. Hemostatic Effect: It is a hydrotherapeutic measure to stop bleeding from vessels. The method is useful in capillary oozing rather than large vessel bleeding. It can be of two types:

1. **Direct Hemostatic effect**
2. **Indirect Hemostatic effect**

Temperature of application:

Very hot (140°– 160°F)

Very cold (32° -40°F)

Mode of application:

- Hot douche
- Hot compress
- Jet of hot steam
- Ice compress
- Ether or Rhigolene spray

1. **Direct Hemostatic effect:** Direct application is done at the bleeding area or at the trunk of an artery(ice collar or cravat or epistaxis**.)** There are various other methods found beneficial.

   Eg: **Epistaxis:** Hot nasal douche**,** Sponging the face with very hot water.

   Menorrhagia: Hot vaginal douche, hot uterine irrigation

   Post partum hemorrhage: hot uterine irrigation

   Vesicle hemorrhage: Hot bladder irrigation.

2. **Indirect Hemostatic effect:** This effect is produced through the indirect application away from the bleeding site through reflex action.

   > Eg**: Epistaxis:** Placing the hands in ice water, ice application to the cervical & upper dorsal portion of the spine. placing the feet in cold water(can be utilized with other methods)

   > **Pulmonary Hemorrhage:** Cold compress to the chest & very hot fomentation between the shoulder blades covering lower cervical & upper dorsal area.

   Ice application to the nostrils (causes pulmonary vessel contraction – Brown Sequard)

> **Hemorrhage from the stomach:** Swallowing of ice cubes

  Ice compress over the epigastrium.

> **Apoplexy:** Ice cap or ice compress to the head, face and neck

> **Uterine hemorrhage:** Short very hot fomentation or hot douche to the thighs and spine.

  Ice bag over the lower abdomen with a hot vaginal douche.

  Short hot douche to the lumbar region, inner surface of the thighs & soles of the foot.

  Prolonged cold applications (55° - 75°F) to the lumbar region, inner surface of the thighs & soles of the foot.

b. Cardiac Excitants: These applications stimulate the activity of the heart. Water is a powerful means for this purpose.

With prolonged cold applications initial quickening of heart activity is followed by slowing down & energizing its function. Prolonged hot applications slow down the function initially followed by quickening & weakening the heart function.

Applications that tonify the heart / Cardiac tonics:

- Short very hot fomentation over the heart
- Very hot or very cold compress over the chest and trunk or to other larger areas
- Very short cold application to the face and chest, Eg: sprinkling cold water on the face of a fainting person.
- Ice bag or ice compress over the heart area: continuous application is contra indicated. Ice cold application for half an hour three times a day or once in 2 to three hours can be given according to the patient's condition. Friction is given on the cooled areas to maintain the blood flow & nerve sensibility.
- Cold compress (60° to 70°F) over the chest area.
- Cold applications to the rectal and gastric mucous membrane excite the cardiac & pulmonary circulation.
- Very short hot bath
- Short hot blanket pack
- Hot & cold immersion bath
- Moderate dry friction
- Hot & Cold applications to the spine
- Hot water drinking
- Hot enema

Note: Comparing the effects of alcohol, digitalis & water on cardiac function

- Alcohol reduces the work & working power of the heart

- Digitalis increases the work & working power of the heart

- Cold water reduces the work & increases the working power.

c. Uterine Excitation: These are the measures which stimulate uterine contraction & enhance the circulation of ovaries & uterus thus improving their nutrition & function.

Hydriatic applications: Measures to stimulate uterine contraction in delayed labor are:

- Cold application to the lower abdomen

- Short & sudden cold application to the mammary glands

- Hot vaginal douche

- Alternate hot & cold applications to the breast & lower abdomen

Measures to enhance uterine & ovarian circulation in Amenorrhoea:

- Short cold douche to the lumbar region

d. Vesicle Excitation: These are the measures that stimulate the contraction of the urinary bladder.

Hydriatic application:

- Cold douche to the feet & over the area of bladder in case of motor insufficiency of the bladder.

Contra indication: Urine retention due to obstruction.

e. Peristaltic Excitation: These are the measures that stimulate the intestinal activity.

Hydriatic application:

- Hot enema
- Cold enema
- Graduated enema
- Cold douche
- Alternate douche
- Applications over the loins & entire abdomen mainly around the umbilicus
- Hot &cold rectal douche

Stimulation of the gastric motility:

- Cold application to the epigastrium or to the dorsal spine
- Sipping of cold water
- Ice bag application over the epigastrium half an hour before food.

2. SECONDARY EXCITANT EFFFECTS (REACTION):

These are the reaction effects. Secondary excitation effect is obtained by cold applications rather than hot applications. Since hot applications are sedative or atonic in nature. Heat is applied in alternate applications to intensify the effect of cold and to produce its own excitation.

There are two types of secondary excitation effects according to the type of application.

1. General secondary excitant effects

2. Local secondary excitant effects

1. General secondary excitant effects:

A short very cold application is an excitant measure. The excitation effect is amplified with addition of percussion effect in douche. Practically there are three subtypes of general secondary excitant effects.

a. Restorative

b. Tonic

c. Calorific

a. Restorative Effect: The applications which restore the energy when exhausted or having a refreshing effect are restorative in nature.

Hydriatic applications:

- Single short application of cold water as douche, affusion, rubbing wet sheet or immersion.

- Cold water application to face, head, neck & spine.
- General cold friction
- Cold arm & foot bath
- Short hot bath (2 to 4 min, at 104°to 110°F) followed by cold friction (in case of collapse due to fever)

Indications:

- Extreme exhaustion
- After vigorous exercise
- Collapse due to fever

Note: Cold bath can be given when the surface is hot & dry or with perspiration.

Precautions: A general cold bath should not be given

- when the body surface is cold, blue and covered with cold perspiration
- during severe fatigue due to any cause
- When the patient has infectious fever
- When patient has chills.

b. Tonic Effect: Applications which increase the vital activity to restore the normal tone or conditions of the body. Circulation, nutrition and other bodily functions are enhanced. Strong tonics are the strong excitants. Cold water is an excellent tonic when applied regularly.

Cold water application has an advantage over medicinal tonics since cold water stimulates nervous activity without putting extra burden on any organ or modifying its function.

Definition of tonic according to Trousseau:

Tonic is an agent having for its object to give tone to the tissues, to restore the function of nutrition & assimilation and to increase the vital resistance.

Modern Definition: An agent which when systematically employed aids in the restoration of normal tissue activities both constructive & destructive, thereby promoting a renewal of the body and recuperation of its forces and an increase of vital resistance.

Hydriatic applications:.

- **All short cold applications (Most pronounced effect with repetition of very short very cold bath**

    a. **With percutient effect (douche):** rain douche, horizontal jet, spinal douche, circle douche, massage douche, pail douche or affusion, scotch douche, alternate douche, percussion douche.

    b. **Without percutient effect (with strong friction):** wet sheet rub, towel rub, cold friction, wet hand rub, plunge bath, sitz bath, full immersion bath

Short cold applications produce tonic effect. This can be enhanced by the application of douche in any form. In Douche mechanical effect is added to the thermic effect of cold application to strengthen the reaction. Temperature of application should be below 90°F to produce the tonic effect. Tonic applications can be sedative if prolonged. This is noticed by reducing of rectal temperature few tenths of a degree. Changing over of tonic effects to sedative effects depends upon the course of treatment & condition & vulnerability of the patient.

Mechanism: Repeating the excitant measures produces tonic effect. These cold applications fill the skin blood vessels as a tonic reaction. On repeating the procedure daily vascular activity in the skin is increased and it relieves inner congestion.

Indications: Anemia, Exhaustion, hysteria, insomnia, obesity, exopthalmic goiter, convalescence from fever, hypochondria, nervous dyspepsia, melancholia, acute infectious fever.

Precautions:

1. Very weak persons have strong need for tonic measures. Since they cannot tolerate cold applications, initially milder applications have to be given in the form of

   - Cold wet hand rub
   - Cold friction

- Salt glow
- Alternate hot & cold applications to the spine
- Dry friction
- Short hot bath before the cold applications

2. In the beginning of tonic applications fatigue is experienced by weak patients. This is due to their weak vitality which is unable to support the loss of body heat & nervous energy. It is indicated by chillness & other nervous symptoms. Care must be taken not to weaken the patient.

3. Short cold application to chest produces cough, oppression & distress due to the influence of cold on respiratory system. Care should be taken while treating the cases of asthma,, dyspnea and cardiac weakness.

4. Avoid percutient (cold douche) applications in following conditions:

   - Over the chest area especially in pulmonary congestion or hypersensitivity of pulmonary area.
   - Over the stomach, loin & abdomen in hyperpepsia, stomach ulcer, bleeding from the bowel, menorrhagia or metrorrhagia.

5. Great care must be taken when treating very weak patients (convalescence from fever, wasting disease, severe hemorrhage).

6. Nervous or neurasthenic patients should be treated with hot bath(3 to 10 min.) in the form of electric light or vapor bath followed by cold application. Cold can be applied at -

   ✓ 65° to 70°F for 4 to 6 seconds.

   ✓ 75° to 80° F for 10 to 20 seconds.

Note:

1. Scotch douche is very effective in the treatment of weak & anemic patient.

2. Tonic applications for cerebral congestion: cold application to the legs in the form of broken douche, rubbing wet sheet, cold friction. Repeatation of the application daily produces pronounced effects.

3. In cases of Rheumatism moderate cold application should be preceded by a hot application so as to produce perspiration. Cold application is avoided on the painful joints.

c. Calorific Effects: These applications stimulate the heat production in the body. All the restorative & tonic applications produce calorific effects.

Hydriatic applications: Short cold immersion bath, (20 sec. to 2 minutes), Cold douche with less pressure, cold affusion, wet sheet pack prolonged till the beginning of 4th stage (Sweating Stage).

2. Local Secondary Excitant Effects: Water applications which affect the function of an organ or system are local secondary excitants. They are classified as follows:

1. Sudorific a) Spoliative b)Eliminative
2. Expectorant
3. Cholagogic
4. Peptogenic
5. Emmenagogic
6. Hemostatic
7. Revulsive
8. Derivative
9. Resolutive
10. Alterative
11. Calorific

1. Sudorific Effects: Hydriatic applications which stimulate perspiration are called as sudorific.

Hydriatic applications:

- Electric light bath
- Turkish bath
- Russian bath
- Hot air bath
- Vapor bath

- Hot full bath
- Wet sheet pack
- Dry pack
- Hot douche
- Vapor Douche
- Hot blanket pack
- Hot sitz bath
- Hot water drinking
- Hot enema
- Hot fomentation to the spine
- Sun bath

Sweating at a local area can be produced by circumscribed hot applications or by preventing heat loss through warm or impervious coverings.

Note: Electric light bath is the most effective means of producing sweating within 3 to 5 minutes.

Dry pack induces sweating very slowly after one & half an hour to two hours of application.

a. **Spoliative Effect:** Hydriatic applications which increase the oxidation & catabolism in the body, remove serous deposits from the tissues (anasarca, pleural effusion). They have a tendency for weight reduction.

Hydriatic measure:

- Hot application followed by a short general cold application. Cold application(50 - 60°F for 5 to 20 seconds) is given in the form of cold shower bath, cold horizontal douche or an affusion.

- Electric light bath

Indications: Obesity, anasarca, pleural effusion, Bright's disease, dropsy due to anemia, dropsy due to renal diseases, jaundice, aiding in the reduction of hernia or dislocated limb, pluritic adhesions, migraine, gastric neurasthenia, Chronic rheumatism, Chronic peritonitis, sciatica.

Precautions:

- Care has to be taken while applying this measure for cases of dropsy due to cardiac conditions. Extremes of temperature have to be avoided.

- Sweating bath has to be avoided in condition of diabetes with emaciation.

- In conditions of painful skin eruptions, furuncles etc avoid Turkish or dry air bath as they irritate the skin & wet sheet pack as it is extremely exciting. Sweating bath can be given in the form of vapor bath, Russian bath, hot water bath & electric light bath.

- Hot applications aimed at weight reduction should not be prolonged and it should be followed by intense cold application.

Note:

- In chronic renal conditions neutral bath (92° - 95°F) & effervescent bath is more effective. (Neutral bath excites the renal activity)

- Electric light bath is the best sweating measure in cases of Bright's disease since the skin function is stimulated to greater extent with the short application. Exposing the patient to the highly heated atmosphere as in Russian & Turkish bath is also avoided in this bath.

- Sweating baths induce general muscle relaxation & expands the white fibrous tissue which is the component of ligaments. This fact is made use in reducing hernia & dislocated joints.

b. Eliminative Effect: Stimulation of excretion through the kidney, skin & lungs.

Sweating baths can be given to enhance the elimination of metabolic waste from the body. But this measure is useful only in special conditions when the renal function is reduced due to the diseases of the kidney or there is chronic toxemia due to retained tissue poisons.

Hydriatic applications: Hot blanket pack or other sweating baths, electric light bath.

Sweating bath in conditions of toxemia should not be extended & it must be succeeded by short cold applications.

Indications: Bright's disease, gastric neurasthenia, migraine, jaundice, exudates, stiff & swollen joints in Rheumatism, peuritic adhesions, chronic peritonitis, sciatica.

painful eruptions of the skin, furuncles in these conditions vapor bath, Russian bath, hot water bath or electric light bath is recommended instead of Turkish or dry air bath.

2. Expectorant effect: Hydriatic applications that increase the secretions of the mucus membrane lining the airways & relieve congestion in the chest.

Mucous membrane closely resembles skin in its structure & function. Therefore applications which increase the skin activity also increase the activity of mucus membrane.

Hydriatic measures: Russian bath, vapor bath, steam inhalation, chest pack, hot water drinking

Indications: Cold, cough, asthma, affections of throat, ear & nose.

3. Diuretic Effect: Hydriatic applications which increase the activity of the kidney.

Hydriatic measures: A short cold douche to the loins, Cold douche to the lower part of the sternum, heating trunk pack (middle & lower trunk), Fomentation to the lumbar area.

Indications: Renal calculi, Renal insufficiency due to various causes.

4. Cholagogic Effect: Hydriatic applications that stimulate the activity of liver.

Hydriatic applications: Cold horizontal jet over the epigastrium & right hypochondrium with considerable pressure, alternate douche.

For congestion & pain: hot or scotch fan douche without pressure, hot douche or fomentation followed with wet girdle pack, in weak patients fomentation followed by heating compress.

Indications: Infectious jaundice, gall stones, acute congestion & inflammation of liver.

5. Peptogenic Effect: Hydriatic applications that stimulate the secretions of the stomach.

Hydriatic applications:

Hypopepsia: Cold horizontal douche (50° to 70°F) over the area of stomach with pressure (20 to 30 lbs), alternate douche, cold percussion douche, circle douche, ice bag over the stomach for an hour before food, fomentation over the stomach for 1- 2 hours after food.

Antipeptogenic measures for hyperpepsia: applications given just before food and continued for one to two hours afterwards. Eg: hot douche over the stomach, heating trunk compress, hot & heating trunk pack.

6. Emmenagogic Effect: Hydriatic applications that stimulate the menstrual function are emmenogogic in nature.

Hydriatic applications: Cold horizontal jet or spray to the loins (50° to 70° F for 2 to 10 secs with the pressure 20 to 40 lbs), Prolonged hot foot bath(100° to 104°F), hot sitz bbath (100° to 104°F), hot enema (105°F), hot immersion bath, tonic hip pack daily in between the periods, hot hip pack(110°F for 10 to15 mins).

7. Revulsive Effect: Hydriatic applications that cause strong circulatory effect with revulsion of the blood flow to the desired area.

Hydriatic applications:

Revulsive measure to relieve superficial anemia:

Short cold application followed by intense & prolonged rubbing, Cold percussion douche (at 20° to 60°F for 4 to 10 secs), hot & cold compress, heating compress preceded by fomentation or rubbing of the parts, fomentation at 104° to 106°F for 15 to 20 mins.

Revulsive measure to relieve anemia in deep visceras:

General cold douche (at 80°F for 30 to60 secs), shallow bath (80° to 85° F for 5 to 6 minutes), tonic half pack, cold friction, wet sheet rub.

For amenorrhoea: Ice bag & ice compress to the spine, very cold lumbar douche, cold douche to the hypogastrium & inner surface of the thighs, tonic pelvic pack. The effect can be enhanced by supplementing these measures with vaginal irrigation at 110°F for 10 min or 80°F for one min.

Indications: Renal insufficiency, hepatic inactivity, amenorrhoea, enteroptosis, nephroptosis, gastroptosis, atony of pelvic organs.

Revulsive measures to relieve deep congestion:

Very hot fomentation of hot douche to the lumbar spine & inner thighs(pelvic congestion), fomentation followed by heating spinal compress protected with a flannel(spinal congestion), alternate hot & cold compress to related skin area followed by heating compress protected by a flannel (deep passive congestion), very hot (115° to 130° F) application to the abdomen (to relieve visceral pain),

Indications: infectious jaundice, Splenic & hepatic congestion, inflammation of the gastroduodenum & intestines, menorrhagia, subinvolution of the uterus, hemorrhoids, congestion of the prostate, inflammation of the rectum, bladder.

Note:

- ❖ Revulsive effects are produced by very cold, cold, cool, hot or very hot applications. Neutral or warm applications do not produce these effects as they cannot stimulate the nervous activity.

- ❖ High temperature & prolonged application with hot produces intense revulsive effects.

- ❖ Lower temperature & percussion effect with the cold application produces intense revulsive effect
- ❖ Greater temperature difference between the heat & cold in combined applications produces intense revulsive effects.
- ❖ Revulsion is the best method to produce analgesic effect.
- ❖ To obtain revulsive effect circulatory reaction has to be facilitated and thermic reaction has to be avoided.

8. Derivative effect: Drawing the blood or lymph from one part to another.i.e.Relieving the congestion of an organ by deriving the blood to a distant area. Thermic reaction need not be suppressed to produce this effect.

Hydriatic applications:

Local derivative effects: hot leg bath, hot sitz, short cold sitz, rubbing sitz, leg pack, half pack, hot, cold or alternate douche to the legs or arms, cold friction, rubbing shallow pelvic pack, heating abdominal compress.

General derivative effects: wet sheet pack, rubbing wet sheet, general cold friction.

Indications: Insomnia, pulmonary congestion or hemorrhage, apoplexy, acute mania, cerebral congestion.

9. Resolvent Effect: Applications that stimulate the absorption of exudates from joints, muscles & tendons.

Hydriatic applications: alternate douche, fomentation followed by heating compress, alternate hot & cold compress, alternate pail douche(15 sec each).

To produce analgesic effect hot application can be prolonged eg: hot - 60 secs & cold – 15 secs or hot – 2 min & cold – 15 secs.

10. Alterative Effect: An agitation, change or a disturbance produced through the reflex activities initiated in the body on application of water.

Hydriatic applications: Cold douche, alternate douche, wet sheet pack, Immersion bath, sweating baths, hepatic douche, splenic douche, general hot & cold applications.

More pronounced alterative effects will be produced by cold applications with strong percussion. Percussion douche & massage douche produce powerful general alterative effects.

Indications: Refractory cases of malarial infection, chronic neuroses, neuralgias, headache, neurasthenia.

11. Calorific Effects: Applications that stimulate the heat production in the body are calorific in nature.

Hydriatic applications: Heating compress, local cold friction, local cold immersion, prolonged hot application, local hot air bath, local vapor bath, local electric light bath.

Indication: To stimulate the local activity of any part, to prepare the skin for cold applications.

SEDATIVE EFFECTS: Moderating the abnormally increased activity of an organ or set of organs is called as sedative or depressant effect. The agent that induces this change is called sedative agent. Sedative effects can be immediate or remote.

Classification: There are 3 types of sedative effects:-

1. Sedative of the Circulatory system
2. Sedative of the Nervous system
3. Sedative of the metabolic activity
4. Secretory Sedatives

1. Sedative of the Circulatory system:

1. **Antiphlogistic a.Vascular, b. Cardiac**
2. **Hemostatic**

2. Sedative of the Nervous system:

1. **Hypnotic**
2. **Calmative**
3. **Antispasmodic**
4. **Analgesic**
5. **Anesthetic**

3. Sedative of the metabolic activity:

1. **Antithermic**
2. **Anti pyretic**

Means of producing sedative effects:

1. By cold water applications: a). Tonic applications methodically applied to lengthen the duration(remote effect) b). by prolonged applications below 92°F (immediate effect)
2. By warm or hot water applications: a). Short hot applications b). Prolonged neutral applications.

Note:

> **Full immersion bath or neutral bath (92 -97°F) produces direct & immediate sedative effects.**

> **Antiphlogistic, hemostatic, anesthetic & analgesic measures are given for local effects.**

> **Atithermic & antipyretic measures are given for general effects.**

Sedatives of the circulatory system:

Reaction following a cold application is tonic in nature, therefore reaction has to be suppressed to produce a sedative effect. General points to be considered are:

a. Prolonging cold application
b. Avoiding friction & percussion in the application.

1. Antiphlogistic effects: Hydriatic applications which suppress or reduce the local acute congestion or inflammation are called as antiphlogistic.

Indications: boil, acute joint inflammation, pneumonia, pleurisy, peritonitis, phlebitis, erythema.

Hydriatic measures with indications:

a. Cardiac insufficiency or valvular incompetency – cold compress to the precordium for half an hour three times a day. Neutral bath with the friction to energize the peripheral heart.

b. Hepatic sclerosis causing congestion of the organ – broken douche to the lower half of the right chest (60°F), alternate hepatic douche (100° to 60 °F).

c. Congestive headache – to relieve vasospasm in the legs & feet following measures can be given: scotch douche, prolonged hot leg or foot bath, heating pack to the legs, fomentation to the abdomen followed by heating abdominal compress.

d. For moving the stagnated blood in different clinical conditions prolonged cold compress (60° -70°F), alternate hot & cold applications, very hot compress or douche are given. These measures increase the tone of the vessels in the affected area.

e. Prevention of inflammation in lacerated wounds or burns: Prolonged immersion of a part (95° to 97°F) repeating for several days as per the requirement.

f. Fever: Tepid sponging & evaporating compress, neutral bath at 92° to 95°F for 20 min. Friction during or after the bath or exercise after the bath must be avoided.

2. Hemostatic effect: Sedative effect of cold can be utilized for checking bleeding. Very hot & very cold applications can be used for this purpose. Care should be taken to control reaction effect with the cold applications.

Hydriatic measures with indications:

a. Bleeding wound, epistaxis – Ice application

b. Hemorrhage from the stomach – swallowing of ice pills

c. Hemorrhage from the kidney – Ice pack to the loins

d. Hemorrhage from the bowels - Ice bag or compress to the abdomen.

e. Uterine hemorrhage – Ice cold compress to the vulva & perineum, water application to the uterine cavity through a hollow metal sound (Dr. J. H. Kellogg).

Sedatives of the nervous system: Sedative measures of the circulatory system also have the same effect on nervous system. Practically it is difficult to distinguish circulatory & nerve sedatives. Sedation of the nervous system is caused by the lessening of the activity in the cerebrospinal nerves.

Hypnotic or general sedative effect:

Hydriatic applications: Warm bath (92° to 97°F) for 30 min. to two hours., broken jet (85° to92°F) for three minutes, ice cap or cold compress to the head, evaporating head cap, revulsive compress, hot & cold sponging, alternate hot & cold pour, alternate hot & cold douche moist girdle or heating compress over the abdomen at night(insomnia).

Local Analgesic effects:

Hydriatic applications

a. Pain with acute inflammation –Prolonged cold compress (60 to 70°F), ice pack, evaporating compress. After the acute stage application of fomentation (10 to15min.) in between 2 to 6 hours.

b. Chronic pain: Revulsive measures.

c. Acute & chronic pain: Derivative measures.

d. Prolonged hot applications can be given in any painful conditions, interrupt it with a tepid or cold compress every hour for about half a minute.

Prolonged hot applications are avoided in painful conditions of head & eyes.

Indications:

a. Pleurisy, gastralgia, hepatic or renal colic - Very hot fomentation(140 to 160°F).

b. Intestinal colic, enteralgia, renal & hepatic colic, pain due to hyperesthesia of abdominal ganglia – Fomentation, hot enema.

c. Enteritis, colitis, peritonitis(pain due to inflammation) - Very hot fomentation for 15 to 20 min. followed by cold compress for one to two hours and then renewal of fomentation.

d. Pain of hemorrhoids & rectal ulcer – fomentation over the local area, very hot sitz bath.

e. Chronic pelvic pain –Short (3 to 5 min.) very hot sitz bath112° to 120°F) followed by immediate dash of cold water on hips.

f. Sciatica or other neuralgic pain - Revulsive application i.e. very hot fomentation for 15 to 20 min. followed by very cold compress (well dried) to 30 to 60 sec.or cold friction., scotch douche.

g. Congestive headache - ice bag or compress to the head, neck & face.

h. Pain due to sprain & bruises – very hot fomentation(two to three hours) followed by cold compress or ice bag at intervals (15 min.)

i. Pain due to inflamed eyelids – very thin cold compress kept cold by fanning.

j. Pain of the eye ball due to different causes – very hot thin compress (3 to 5 min) followed by cold compress (15 to 30 sec.)

Anesthetic Effect: Lowering skin temperature few degrees below the normal body temperature abolishes its sensibility. Therefore benumbing effect is seen. Ice application, freezing mixture of salt & ice, an ether or rhygolene spray are some of the measures to produce anesthetic effect. Practical utility of this effect of water in modern days is limited.

Antispasmodic Effect:

Hydriatic applications with indications:

a. Hysteria, nervous agitation, insomnia - Neutral Immersion bath for 15 min to an hour or more.

b. Constipation due to contraction of the colon or anus, gall stones, renal colic - hot fomentation, hot sitz bath, hot enema

c. Local antispasmodic effect for different conditions - neutral douche, warm compress, neutral pour, neutral spinal douche without pressure, spinal pour.

Sedatives of the metabolic activity:

1. Antithermic Effects: Hydriatic application which abstracts heat from the body.

General principles of hydriatic applications in reducing temperature:

1. Greater the difference between the body temperature & that of water application more pronounced will be the effect.

2. Application should be prolonged.

3. Percussion is avoided in all applications.

4. Friction is given during the cold bath.

Hydriatic applications:

a. Wet sheet pack (30 min) renewed every 5 to 8 min. (Winternitz)

b. Graduated or brand bath followed by abdominal or trunk compress renewed every half an hour.

c. Water drinking

d. Enema

e. Cooling pack

2. Antipyretic Effects: Hydriatic application which abstracts heat and reduces heat production is antipyretic in nature. Cold and hot water applications produce antipyretic effect when systematically employed. Raise of body temperature in fevers is due to following reasons:

1. Increased heat production

2. Reduced heat elimination

3. Increased heat production & Reduced heat elimination.

4. Other disturbances in heat regulating centres.

Indications of fever due to increased heat production:

a. Flushed face with full pulse

b. Warm moist skin

c. Hot dry skin

Indications of fever due to decreased heat elimination:

a. Cold dry skin

b. Cold moist skin

c. Goose flesh appearance

d. Bluish discoloration of the skin

e. Chills

f. Shivering

Antipyretic hydriatic applications:

1. Cold or tepid affusion: Warm affusions(87° to 97°F) are more effective than cold affusions in fever (Currie).

2. Cold immersion bath or Brand bath

3. Cold friction bath: Rate of heat elimination is significantly increased with friction during the bath (Winternitz).

4. Tepid or neutral bath (92° to 95°F)

5. Graduated bath

6. Cooling wet sheet pack

7. Cold shower pack

8. The cold compress

9. Cold sponge bath

10. The wet towel rub

11. Cold wet friction

12. Cold evaporating sheet

13. Hot evaporating sheet

14. Hot sponge bath

15. Hot Blanket pack given for 3 to 10 min. Indicated in high temperatures with reduced heat elimination.

16. Fomentation to the back or alternate hot and cold compress to the spine.

17. Fomentation to the abdomen: when patient has chills & shivering.

18. Hot & cold bath: Hot bath for 3 mins followed by bath at 95°F then gradual reduction of temperature to 80°F during 5 to 15 min. effectively reduces the temperature in fevers than Brand bath **(Vinaj)**.

   Hot spray (one min.) followed by short cold spray better to reduce temperature in fever than cold spray alone **(Pfluger)**.

19. Cold application to the head, heart, spine & abdomen: Prolonged ice application or ice water coil over the heart lowers blood temperature & thereby reduces the general temperature (Winternitz).

   Ice bag to the spine (Neale).

20. Cold air bath: Breathing cold air, exposing the skin to cold air reduces the tempeture in fever.

21. Graduated compress

22. Water drinking: Drinking two to three pints of cold water (40°F) within 10 min. reduces temperature from 1.5° to2° F (John Hancock)

23. Tepid or cold enema

24. Partial cold application: Local inflammation (Appendicitis, pneumonia, pleurisy, peritonitis, acute arthritis, otitis media etc) causing fever can be treated with cold circumscribed applications to the affected area.

Hydriatic applications for increased heat production & Heat elimination:

1. Graduated bath

2. Cooling wet sheet pack

3. The brand bath or cold friction bath

4. Prolonged tepid immersion bath

5. Cold immersion bath followed by short hot immersion, affusion or sprinkling

6. Tepid affusion
7. Cold affusion
8. The shower pack
9. Cold compress
10. Graduated compress
11. Evaporating sheet
12. Cold to head and neck
13. Cold to spine
14. Cold to abdomen
15. Cold over heart
16. Cold irrigation
17. Tepid or cold enema
18. Cold water drinking (this measure has to be combined with all the above hydriatic applications)
19. Cold air bath

Hydriatic application for reduced heat elimination or no increase in the heat elimination:

Following are the measures indicated during fever and when cold is contraindicated:

1. Hot bath (2 to 3 min.) followed by cold bath (1min.) with friction.
2. Hot blanket pack

3. Hot evaporating sheet

4. Hot sponge bath

5. Fomentation to the back

6. Fomentation to the abdomen, followed by cold enema

7. Fomentation to the back followed by cold wet sheet pack.

8. Hot blanket pack followed by graduated bath

9. Hot blanket pack followed by prolonged tepid bath

10. Hot blanket pack followed by friction

11. Dry friction

12. Cold friction

Precautions & suggestions with regard to application of Antipyretic hydriatic applications:

Cold alone is contraindicated under following conditions:

1. Fever with cold, blue skin, blue lips, gooseflesh appearance, perspiration, general shivering, chillness, aversion to cold applications.

    A short general hot application can be made in such conditions before the cold applications.

2. Application of fomentation to the abdomen will relieve the symptoms of chills & colicky pain during cold enema.

3. Avoid prolonged general cold applications if the fever is due to internal local inflammation (Ovaritis, salpingitis, nephritis, gastritis etc). This is to avoid excess internal congestion which occurs during cold applications & therby further increasing the inflammation.

    Prolonged neutral or tepid applications or local revulsive applications are preferred in these conditions.

4. Avoid too Prolonged hot applications (hot bath, fomentation, hot blanket pack) during fever since it elevates the temperature to dangerous levels. Therefore hot application should be limited to 5 to 10 min.

5. In febrile conditions mild temperatures can be brought down easily than severe ones through hydriatic applications. It is easy to lower the temperatures between 100° to 104°F in febrile patients than when it is very high (104° to 106°F) or near normal (99° to 100°F).

4. Secretory Sedatives: Cold applications lower the temperature of glandular structures and reduce their secretions. Heat stimulates the glandular secretions. Eg: Cold application made on the skin surface reduces profuse sweating. In the same way internal glands can be sedated by neutral or hot (92 - 104°F) applications & excited by cold applications made on the overlying skin surface.

References

1. Rational Hydrotherapy by J.H. Kellogg, M. D

2. A Study of Hydrotherapy and Its Health Benefits Mozhdeh Bahadorfar. International Journal of Research (IJR) Vol-1, Issue-8, September 2014 ISSN 2348-6848.

3. A Review on Hydrotherapy Practices in Ancient India K. J. Sujatha, N. K. Manjunath b Journal of Complementary and Alternative Medical Research 17(1): 22-29, 2022; Article no.JOCAMR.79409 ISSN: 2456-6276.

4. Comparative Study of the Composition of Sweat from Eccrine and Apocrine Sweat Glands during Exercise and in Heat, Yi-Lang Chen et. al in Int. J. Environ. Res. Public Health 2020, 17, 3377.

5. Nursing Times [online] December 2019 / Vol 115 Issue 12, www.nursingtimes.net

6. Anatomy and Physiology of the Skin, South West Regional Wound Care Program.

7. Physiology of sweat gland function: The roles of sweating and sweat composition in human health,

Lindsay B. Baker, TEMPERATURE 2019, VOL. 6, NO. 3, 211–259 https://doi.org/10.1080/23328940.2019.1632145.

8. Skin innervation: important roles during normal and pathological cutaneous repair, Betty Laverdet et. al, Histol Histopathol (2015) 30: 875-892.

9. Anatomy, Physiology and Pathology notes, www.goldeneggholistic.com

10. John E. Hall, Michael E. Hall, Guyton and Hall Textbook of Medical Physiology,14th ed.pdf.

11. Water: structure and properties. Kim A Sharp, E. R. Johnson Research Foundation, University of Pennsylvania, USA.

12. Hydrotherapy: Historical landmarks of a cure all remedy G. TSOUCALAS et.al, Archives of the Balkan Medical Union September 2015, vol. 50, no. 3, pp. 430-432.

13. Hydrotherapy in Ancient Greece. Nikolaos TSITSIS et. al, Balkan Military Medical Review, Oct - Dec 2013; 16(4): 462 – 466.

www.ingramcontent.com/pod-product-compliance
Lightning Source LLC
Chambersburg PA
CBHW031416150726
47989CB00002B/684